ABC OF HEALTH INFORMATICS

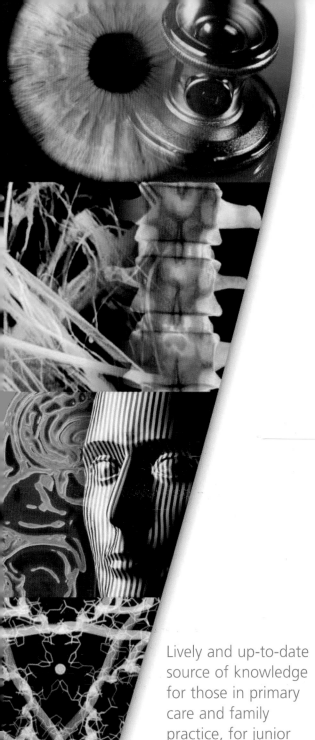
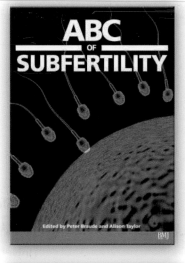
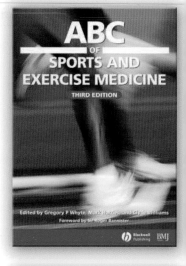
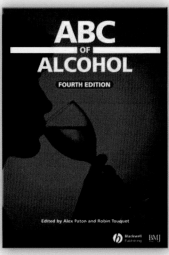
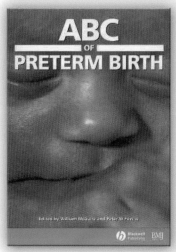
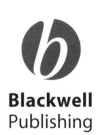
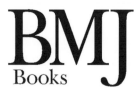

ABC OF HEALTH INFORMATICS

FRANK SULLIVAN
*NHS Tayside professor of research and development in general practice and primary care,
University of Dundee*

JEREMY C WYATT
Professor of health informatics, University of Dundee

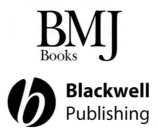

Blackwell Publishing, Inc., 350 Main Street, Malden, Massachusetts 02148-5020, USA
Blackwell Publishing Ltd, 9600 Garsington Road, Oxford OX4 2DQ, UK
Blackwell Publishing Asia Pty Ltd, 550 Swanston Street, Carlton, Victoria 3053, Australia

First published 2006

2 2008

Library of Congress Cataloging-in-Publication Data
Sullivan, Frank (Frank M.)
     ABC of health informatics/Frank Sullivan, Jeremy C. Wyatt.
        p. ; cm.
     Includes bibliographical references and index.
     ISBN: 978-0-7279-1850-5 (alk. paper)
     1. Medical informatics.   I. Wyatt, J. (Jeremy) II. Title.
     [DNLM: 1. Medical Informatics.   W 26.5 S949a 2006]
  R858.S85 2006
  610.28—dc22

2005037646

ISBN: 978 0 7279 1850 5

A catalogue record for this title is available from the British Library

Cover image is courtesy of Mark Garlick/Science Photo Library

Set by BMJ Electronic Production
Printed and bound in Singapore by COS Printers Pte Ltd

Commissioning Editor: Eleanor Lines
Editorial Assistant: Victoria Pittman
Development Editor: Sally Carter/Nick Morgan
Production Controller: Debbie Wyer

For further information on Blackwell Publishing, visit our website:
http://www.blackwellpublishing.com

Contents

Foreword   vii

1   What is health information?   1

2   Is a consultation needed?   4

3   Why is this patient here today?   7

4   How decision support tools help define clinical problems   10

5   How computers can help to share understanding with patients   13

6   How informatics tools help deal with patients' problems   16

7   How computers help make efficient use of consultations   19

8   Referral or follow-up?   22

9   Keeping up: learning in the workplace   25

10 Improving services with informatics tools   29

11 Communication and navigation around the healthcare system   32

12 eHealth and the future: promise or peril?   35

    Glossary   39

    Index   43

Foreword

Information technology is worthy of consideration in its own right as a prime mover of change, and not simply as a means to an end. White's *Medieval Technology and Social Change* is a wonderful and short classic. The author, a distinguished historian, points out that most history is written by priests and politicians, "scribblers" in his words, who are concerned with policy and strategy documents or ideology. However, massive changes are brought about in society by the introduction of technologies that have unforeseen social impacts. For example, the stirrup led to the creation of feudalism; the heavy plough to the manorial system in northern Europe.

We spend a great deal of time agonising about the future of the medical profession and the nature of clinical practice and education, but information technology is a tool that will be as dramatic in its impact as the stirrup or the heavy plough. Often people try to dissociate themselves from information technology and say they are in knowledge management or the information business, but information technology is itself of vital importance and we should be proud to be making the tools.

This collection of essays, from two distinguished and practical clinical academics, gives an excellent introduction to the revolutionary potential of healthcare information technology, the social impact of which will be enormous. We are fortunate today that those who create and develop such tools are, unlike their glorious predecessors, able to write—and to write beautifully. I have great pleasure in recommending this book to readers from all backgrounds as an accessible, comprehensive survey of this revolutionary technology.

Sir JA Muir Gray
Director of Clinical Knowledge, Process and Safety
NHS Connecting for Health

Further reading

White L, Jr. *Medieval technology and social change.* New York: Oxford University Press Inc, 1968.

1 What is health information?

Information is an ethereal commodity. One definition describes it as the data and knowledge that intelligent systems (human and artificial) use to support their decisions. Health informatics helps doctors with their decisions and actions, and improves patient outcomes by making better use of information—making more efficient the way patient data and medical knowledge is captured, processed, communicated, and applied. These challenges have become more important since the internet made access to medical information easier for patients.

This ABC focuses on information handling during routine clinical tasks, using scenarios based on Pendleton's seven-stage consultation model (see box opposite). The chapters cover wider issues arising from, and extending beyond, the immediate consultation (see box below). Questions on clinical information that often arise in clinical and reflective practice are dealt with, but discussion of specific computer systems is avoided.

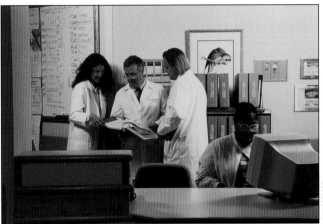

JOHN GREIM/SPL

Some questions on clinical information

Medical record keeping
- What records to keep?
- In what format?
- What data to enter, and how?
- How to store records, and for how long?
- With whom to share the record?

How to use the information records contain
- To manage my patients?
- To audit and improve my service?
- To support my research?
- To feed another information system?

How to communicate with my colleagues and patients
- Face to face?
- On paper?
- Using the internet?

Clinical knowledge sources
- What knowledge sources are out there, and how to select them?
- How to use these sources to answer my own, and my team's, clinical questions?
- How to keep knowledge and skills up to date?
- How to use knowledge to improve my own, and my team's, clinical practice?

Pendleton's consultation model, adapted for ABC series

- Discover the reason for the patient's attendance
- Consider other problems
- Achieve a shared understanding of the problems with the patient
- With the patient, choose an appropriate action for each problem
- Involve the patient in planning their management
- Make effective use of the consultation
- Establish or maintain a relationship with the patient

Ms Smith is a 58 year old florist with a 15 year history of renal impairment caused by childhood pyelonephritis who is experiencing tiredness and muscle cramps. She has sought medical attention for similar problems in the past, and is considering doing so again

---

Capturing and using information

Consider the different forms that information can take, where each form comes from, its cost, and how to assess the quality of the information. These issues arise during a general practitioner's (Dr McKay) encounter with Ms Smith.

Dr McKay applies her own clinical knowledge and skill, perhaps augmented by a textbook or other knowledge source, to capture relevant data from Ms Smith. Dr McKay browses Ms Smith's record to check her medical history. She updates the record and either takes action herself, or telephones a consultant nephrologist (Dr Jones), who suggests 1α-hydroxy cholecalciferol 0.5 µg daily for Ms Smith. Dr McKay then follows up the telephone conversation with the consultant by issuing an electronic prescription. The prescription transfers through a secure local network to Ms Smith's usual pharmacist

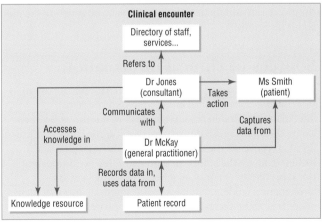

Information flows in a clinical environment

along with a formal online outpatient referral request. Dr Jones checks a hospital phone directory on the web before referring Ms Smith to the dietician for a low calcium diet. Ms Smith is kept informed of these developments by telephone before her appointment the next week.

Representing, interpreting and displaying information

When Dr McKay reads Ms Smith's patient record what she sees on the page is not actually information, but a representation of it. A "real" item of information, such as the fact that Ms Smith has hypercalcaemia, is distinct from how that item is represented in an information system (for example, by selecting Ms Smith's record and writing "Hypercalcaemia," or choosing a Read code that updates Ms Smith's computer-based record). The real information is also distinct from a person's interpretation of it, which might resemble a fragment in a stream of consciousness, "Remember to check on Ms Smith—calcium problem back again." These distinctions reflect common sense and semiotic theory: real things only exist in the physical world, and each person interprets them in private and associates their own images with them.

Back in the clinical world, the lesson is that we should capture and represent each item of information in a form that helps each user—whether human or computer—to find and interpret it. The next time Dr McKay logs into Ms Smith's computer record, although Ms Smith's serum calcium may be represented internally in the computer as the real number 2.8, on the computer screen it can be shown as a figure, a red warning icon, a point on a graph showing all her calcium results, or as the words "Severe hypercalcaemia" in an alert. These display formats can all be achieved with a paper record, but it would take more time and effort to annotate abnormal laboratory results with a highlighter pen, graph the values on a paper chart, or write an alert on a Post-it note and place this on the front of Ms Smith's record.

Selecting a format is important because it determines how to represent each item of information in a system, and in turn how each item is captured. When information is captured and represented on paper or film, it is hard to change the order in which each item appears or to display it in other formats. When information is captured and stored on a computer, however, it can be shown in a different order or grouped in different ways. When data is coded and structured, or broken down into simple elements, it can be processed automatically—for example, the computer can add the icon, graph the data, or generate the alert about Ms Smith.

Sources of clinical information

Clinicians use three types of information to support patient care: patient data, medical knowledge, and "directory" information. This description ignores two questions, however: where does the knowledge in a textbook come from, and how do we improve on the methods used to manage patients? Patient data are the source in both cases (see box opposite). Local problems—such as an adverse event or failure to implement a guideline that everyone agrees to apply to their patients—can be picked up by quality improvement activities such as clinical governance. In well organised clinical environments and specialties, a registry is used to capture patient experiences and monitor for adverse outcomes.

Sometimes, however, patient data are used to suggest, or even answer, more general questions—for example, about drug

---

Common sense meets semiotic theory

In her shop, Ms Smith sells a kind of flower that grows on shrubs with prickly stems and serrated leaves. Humans use consistent symbols to represent these things (for example, "rose; roos"). However, each person privately adds their own connotations to these symbols

Some definitions of rose from *Chambers 21st Century Dictionary*
- An erect or climbing thorny shrub that produces large, often fragrant, flowers that may be red, pink, yellow, orange, or white, or combinations of these colours, followed by bright-coloured fleshy fruits
- The national emblem of England
- A light pink, glowing complexion (put the roses back in one's cheeks)
- A perforated nozzle, usually attached to the end of a hose, watering can, or shower head that makes the water come out in a spray

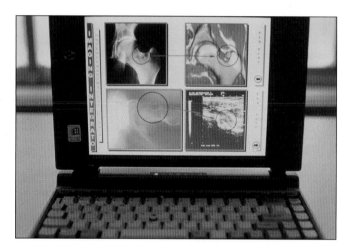

Possible formats to display information include informal or structured text, tables, graphs, sketches, and images. The best format for each item of information depends on who will use it, how they will use it, for what task, and on the formats readily available. With permission from Klaus Gulbrandsen/SPL

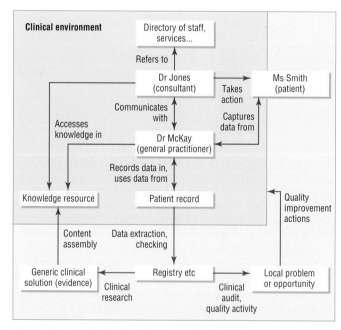

Information flows in clinical and non-clinical environments

effectiveness, disease aetiology, or the accuracy of tests. The results should be high quality, generic evidence that can be safely applied outside the specific clinical environment that is being studied. Often, this evidence is published as if it were the final word. Clinical epidemiology shows us, however, that the results of a single study often differ substantially from the "truth." Well conducted systematic reviews of all rigorous, relevant studies are a better approximation, and are an example of the content assembly methods used to develop good quality knowledge resources.

The costs of information

To a businessman, information must seem the ultimate product: once it is captured, it can be sold any number of times without using up the original supply. Unfortunately for clinicians, each item of information that is captured, processed, and displayed has an associated cost or risk. By choosing to code the current problem as chronic pyelonephritis only (see figure above), Dr McKay fails to record the endocrine dimension with potential loss of explanatory power for others looking at Ms Smith's records. Entering more than one code takes extra time and may cause difficulties in interpretation for secondary use of the data.

Information costs are especially high for data captured by health professionals in the structured, coded representation often required by computerised record systems. If the information is only ever going to be read by humans, it should not be captured as structured data because this will discourage doctors from recording useful free text that computers do not need to "understand"—for example, "Ms Smith is going to Spain for a holiday, her cat died last week." All patient record systems should allow easy entry of such unstructured text (perhaps by voice recognition) to support the human side of medicine, and to help maintain the therapeutic relationship with patients.

Assessing the quality of information

Imagine that Dr Jones is auditing outcomes in his hypercalcaemic patients and wishes to include Ms Smith's data. Is her data of adequate quality for this task?

Information only exists to support decisions and actions: if it fails to do this, it is irrelevant noise. The aims of clinical audit are to understand current practice and suggest appropriate actions for the future. If the data are full of errors or incomplete, refer to patients seen years ago, or cannot be interpreted by the user, they are unlikely to help. More subtly, if useful data items are present—for example, serum calcium—but vital context is omitted, such as serum albumin or current treatment, it is still hard to use the data. Without this context, information is often useless; with it, data collected for one purpose can often, but not always, be used for another.

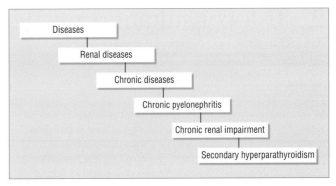

Partial hierarchy of diseases

Quality criteria for patient data

Criterion	How to test it	Comment
Accurate	Comparison with a gold standard source of data—for example, the patient	Technically, validity—does the data item measure what it is meant to? Reliability is a related concept—do two observers agree on the data item?
Complete	Per cent missing data at a given point	Often difficult to estimate without access to multiple sources of information
Timely	Delay from the event the data describes to its availability for use on the information system	Unless data are available at the point they are needed to inform decisions, fulfilling the other criteria is almost worthless
Relevant	Amount that data alter decisions or actions of the user; the impact of leaving an item out of the dataset	Unless data are relevant to information users, they contribute to information overload
Appropriately represented	Degree of structuring and coding of items	Depends on the user of the item and their needs
Relevant detail included	If data are detailed enough to support decisions	Highly dependent on the purpose and confidentiality of the information
Relevant context included	Is there enough context (for example, date patient seen, by whom) to support appropriate interpretation of data?	A key issue, only partially solved in current electronic patient records

Glossaries for informatics terms

- Coiera E. *Guide to health informatics.* 2nd ed. London: Hodder Arnold, 2003. www.coiera.com/glossary.htm (accessed 26 August 2005)
- Wyatt JC, Liu J. Basic concepts in medical informatics. http://jech.bmjjournals.com/cgi/content/full/56/11/808 (accessed 26 August 2005)

Further reading

- Hersh W. What is Medical Informatics? www.ohsu.edu/dmice/whatis/index.shtml (accessed 26 August 2005)
- Pendleton D, Schofield T, Tate P, Havelock P. *The consultation: an approach to learning and teaching.* Oxford: Oxford University Press, 1987
- Nygren E, Wyatt JC, Wright P. Medical records 2: helping clinicians find information and avoid delays. *Lancet* 1998;352:1462-6
- Morris AD, Boyle DI, MacAlpine R, Emslie-Smith A, Jung RT, Newton RW, et al. The diabetes audit and research in Tayside Scotland (DARTS) study: electronic record linkage to create a diabetes register. DARTS/MEMO Collaboration. *BMJ* 1997;315:524-8
- Naylor CD. Grey zones of clinical practice: some limits to evidence based medicine. *Lancet* 1995;345:840-2
- Brody H. *Stories of sickness.* Yale: Yale University Press, 1987
- Tanenbaum SJ. What physicians know. *N Engl J Med* 1996.329:1268-71
- van Bemmel JH, Musen MA, eds. *Handbook of medical informatics.* London: Springer, 1997 www.mihandbook.stanford.edu/handbook/home.htm (accessed 26 August 2005)

2 Is a consultation needed?

People with health concerns no longer have to become patients by consulting a health professional. Electronic health (eHealth) tools provide access to many resources that may satisfy their requirements. This article describes ways that patients can investigate health issues before, or instead of, a consultation.

As a professional, Ms Patel (see box opposite) can access health resources on the internet at work and at home. She may subscribe to a mobile internet service provider through her telephone or palmtop computer. Internet access is not restricted to affluent people in western societies. In the United Kingdom, the 2003 national statistics omnibus survey showed that 48% of households have home internet access, and the figures from the United States are even higher (60% of households have access). Internet cafes can be found worldwide, and library services often provide time online for free. The public can pay for "push technologies" from publishers that supply health alerts, but most people search for the information they need.

Using a search engine

Internet search engines are software tools that index and catalogue websites. People with little or no prior knowledge of a subject, but with some experience of searching the internet, often use search engines to begin an inquiry.

If Ms Patel types "breast cancer and family" into a search engine (such as Google), in 0.23 seconds she may be overwhelmed by more than 5 million websites dealing with the topic. She will be helped by the fact that the search engine has sorted each "hit" by the number of other websites to which it is linked. The list is ordered, and so Ms Patel can start near the top of the list by reading the brief descriptions, or she may use "advanced search" options to narrow the initial search. Advanced searches allow specific phrases, languages, and times to be defined. This reduces the hits to a more manageable number. The most popular sites will probably be those whose content matches patients' preferences for appearance, or those that contain the information patients' are looking for. The most popular sites do not necessarily have features that are the markers of quality preferred by health professionals. If the site does not answer patients' questions, it may provide links to other sites that can. Alternatively, patients can return to the search list and start again.

Patient orientated health portals

These are specalised search engines with additional features such as access to frequently asked questions about health or email facilities. Individual clinicians, clinics, practices, hospitals, and health maintenance organisations provide portals to their own and other resources.

National and local health services (for example, the NHS in the UK) often provide access to such resources for patients. These portals may link to specific services provided by that health service, such as lists of local cancer genetics clinics.

Other portals are provided by independent bodies. Many have international links and are funded by charities. They vary in quality. Some are quality assured, and when they are not, tools are available to allow patients to assess the portal.

Patients make sophisticated use of multiple sources of information. In one study, half of the users of the database of

Ms Amulya Patel is a 48 year old accountant whose mother has recently died of breast cancer. Ms Patel wonders about her own level of risk, and uses the internet to search for patient resources

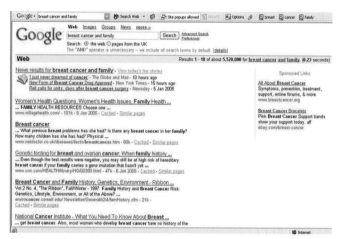

Google search results for "breast cancer and family"

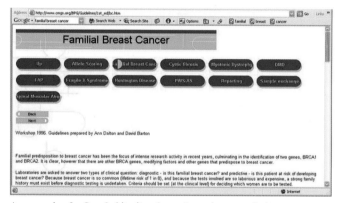

An example of a Google hit—sites chosen by patients usually have immediate facts, such as women have a one in eight lifetime risk of developing cancer

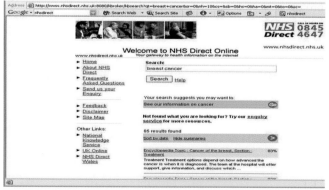

NHS Direct is a health portal aimed at the public

patient experience (DIPEX) who were interested in breast cancer accessed internet resources to obtain second opinions on a range of problems. They sought support and information from patients who had similar issues, obtained information about tests and interventions, and identified questions to ask doctors if necessary.

Many portals link to other websites, and they may direct the person to other resources such as books, multimedia resources, or patient support groups

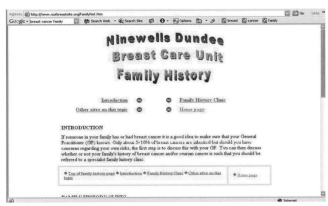

A relevant health service resource accessed through a portal

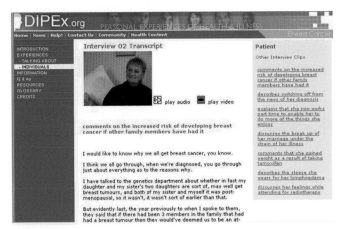

DIPEX allows patients (like Ms Patel) to read, listen, or watch patients facing similar problems to their own

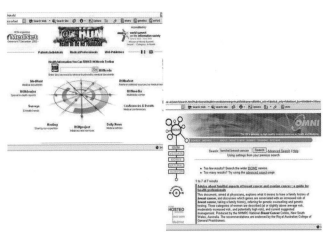

Two examples of quality assured portals

Direct access to medical literature

Some health portals link directly to websites that present medical literature intended for professional use. Patients like those in Ms Patel's situation may have gone straight to such resources because they have heard that they will probably contain the information they are seeking. Ms Patel could access primary data sources, such as the *BMJ* or the *Journal of Medical Genetics,* directly. Sometimes journals provide free access to all their content, others make only article abstracts or brief summaries available.

Most patients will have difficulty in interpreting medical journals (as is the case for many doctors). Risk may be described in absolute or relative terms as percentages, rates, multiples, and over different time periods. Because of the complex nature of the articles and papers in medical journals, many people prefer professional help to translate the information that they have found.

Jargon may make the information resource impenetrable to non-professionals, and some professionals

Mediated access to medical literature

Several journals have patient orientated summaries that highlight one of their recent scientific papers in a broader context and translate the content into a more readable format. The *New England Journal of Medicine* and *JAMA* are notable in this regard, although subscriptions are needed to access many of these services. Therefore, they may be available only if accessed by the health professional on the patient's behalf.

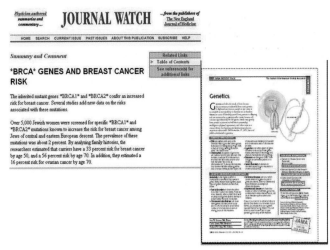

Patient summaries in journals can be helpful

Some clinics make questionnaires and guidelines available on their website, but people can find them difficult to interpret. The questionnaire opposite prompts Ms Patel to ask her relatives about the causes of death of other members of her family. She finds that, in addition to her mother, two maternal aunts had breast cancer.

Examples of familial breast cancer management guidelines

Breast Cancer UK Cancer Family Study Group guidelines for referral and screening mammography*

- One relative with breast cancer diagnosed at <40 years
- Two relatives with breast cancer diagnosed at 40-49 years
- Three relatives with breast cancer who were diagnosed at 50-60 years
- One relative with breast cancer diagnosed at <50 years, and one or more relatives with ovarian cancer diagnosed at any age, or one relative with breast and ovarian cancer

American College of Medical Genetics/New York State Department of Health candidates for consideration for BRCA1 and BRCA2 testing†

- Three or more affected first degree or second degree relatives on the same side of the family, regardless of age at diagnosis, *or*
- <3 Affected relatives, but patient diagnosed at ≤45 years, *or*
- A family member has been identified with a detectable mutation, *or*
- One or more cases of ovarian cancer at any age, and one or more members on same side of family with breast cancer at any age, *or*
- Multiple primary or bilateral breast cancer in patient or one family member, *or*
- Breast cancer in a male patient, or in a male relative, *or*
- Patient is an increased risk for specific mutation(s) because of ethnic background—for example, Ashkenazi Jewish descent—and has one or more relatives with breast cancer or ovarian cancer at any age

*Eccles D, Evans D, Mackay J. Guidelines for managing women with a family history of breast cancer. *J Med Genetics* 2000;37:2-3-9
†American College of Medical Genetics. Genetics susceptibility to breast and ovarian cancer assessment, counselling and testing guidelines, 1999

Teleconsultation

If the person finds an electronic resource that covers their query, then no consultation may be needed. Often, however, general information will need to be supplemented by knowledge of a person's situation. Ms Patel may email her general practitioner or follow a website link to a specialist in the genetics of familial breast cancer. The advantages of email include asynchronous interaction (patients and doctors can submit and receive responses at their convenience), easy exchange of follow-up information, patient education (by attaching leaflets or links to websites), and automatic documentation of consulting behaviour or service requests. Regulation of teleconsultation varies between countries, and guidelines are available. Security and confidentiality issues must be overcome, and there is increasing pressure to do so. Biometric methods, such as logging in using fingerprints or voice recognition, may be a solution in the medium term. Webcams or other video messaging techniques allow real time, albeit virtual, face to face consultations. To provide teleconferencing, doctors may have to alter their daily schedules.

Summary

Before seeing a doctor, Ms Patel found useful information about familial breast cancer. The information prompted her to ask questions of her family, and she found a strong familial history of breast cancer. She sought professional advice. A computer literate person who wants to find out about a health issue may find a satisfactory answer online, but those who become patients will probably need the expertise from doctors that they trust to interpret data for them.

SAMPLE CANCER FAMILY HISTORY QUESTIONNAIRE

- Name
- Date
- Age
- Ethnic Background [Certain ethnic groups have an increased risk for specific kinds of cancer.]

- Do you have any specific concerns about cancer in yourself or your family?

- Do you or any members of your family have a history of cancer?

	Yes/No	Type of Cancer (if known)	Age at Diagnosis (if known)	Living/ Deceased
yourself				
your mother				
your father				
your sisters and brothers				
your half sisters and half brothers				
your children				
your mother's sisters and brothers				
your father's sisters and brothers				
your nieces and nephews				
your mother's parents				
your father's parents				

Risk assessment sheet obtained from the internet

Further reading

- National Statistics Office. Internet access: households and individuals, 2002 www.statistics.gov.uk/pdfdir/inta1202.pdf
- Pagliari C, Sloan D, Gregor P, Sullivan F, Detmer D, Kahan JP, et al. What is eHealth (4): A scoping exercise to map the field. *J Med Internet Res* 2005;7:e9 www.jmir.org/2005/1/e9/ (accessed 6 September 2005)
- Gagliardi A, Jadad AR. Examination of instruments used to rate quality of health information on the internet: chronicle of a voyage with an unclear destination. *BMJ* 2002;324:569-73
- Meric F, Bernstam EV, Mirza NQ, Hunt KK, Ames FC, Ross MI, et al. Breast cancer on the world wide web: cross sectional survey of quality of information and popularity of websites. *BMJ* 2002;324:577-81
- Charnock D, Shepperd S, Needham G, Gann R. DISCERN: an instrument for judging the quality of written consumer health information on treatment choices. *J Epidemiol Community Health* 1999;53:105-11
- Ziebland S, Chapple A, Dumelow C, Evans J, Prinjha S, Rozmovits L. How the internet affects patients' experience of cancer: a qualitative study. *BMJ* 2004;328:564-9
- Gaster B, Knight CL, DeWitt D, Sheffield J, Assefi NP, Buchwald D. Physicians' use of and attitudes towards electronic mail for patient communication. *J Gen Int Med* 2003;18:385-9
- Sands Z. Help for physicians contemplating use of e-mail with patients. *J Am Inf Assoc* 2004;11:268-9
- Finch T, May C, Mair F, Mort M, Gask L. Integrating service development with evaluation in telehealthcare: an ethnographic study. *BMJ* 2003;327:1205-9

3 Why is this patient here today?

Defining the reason for a patient's consultation may seem straightforward, but often deeper consideration is required. Information tools are less important in this phase of the consultation than other phases, but may augment the interpersonal skills of the doctor. At this early stage an open question like "How can I help you today?" and attention to non-verbal cues are more likely to be productive than launching into a closed question and answer session.

If the doctor knows Mr Evans (see box opposite), he will already have noticed the sad expression on the patient's face when he went to the waiting room to call him in to the consultation. The slow, hesitant speech with which Mr Evans talks of his headache is another item of non-verbal information indicating a possible diagnosis of depression.

> **Mr Edward Evans is a 49 year old, recently unemployed, pharmaceutical company representative who presents with headaches. He also has symptoms of early morning wakening and erectile dysfunction**

Diagnostic process

Mr Evans has come to see his general practitioner (GP) because of headaches, sleep disturbance, and sexual difficulties. These problems need to be considered in detail. The symptoms are common in general practice, and most experienced doctors and nurse practitioners will have an approach to assessment with which they are comfortable. Experienced doctors use hypothetico-deductive reasoning methods when assessing patients' problems. An initial clinical feature, headache perhaps, prompts a doctor to recall an "illness script" derived from his or her experience and education that seems to explain a patient's problems. The doctor hypothesises that the diagnosis is, in this case, possibly depression, and tests this hypothesis by asking further questions, examining the patient, or doing laboratory tests to confirm or rule out the diagnosis.

Less experienced doctors may use a checklist or, when an unusual presentation occurs, they may return to inductive reasoning learnt as an undergraduate or trainee. This more exhaustive process involves taking a complete history, carrying out a full systematic examination, and then developing a differential diagnosis list. The process may be made more efficient by using a reference folder that contains checklists describing a clinical examination for headache, for example. These checklists or protocols may be stored on desktop computers or other devices. Another option is to access an information source like the *BMJ*'s 10 minute consultation series, which may provide a framework to assess the problem.

Medical history

Each consultation has been likened to a "single frame in a long running cine film." GPs have repeated opportunities to understand their patients' problems. Until this visit, Dr McKay had not seen Mr Evans for about a year. Then, Mr Evans had been made redundant and was having difficulty sleeping. During the current visit, Dr McKay notes from the electronic record that Mr Evans saw another partner in the practice a month ago for tiredness. In the United Kingdom, almost all of a patient's hospital medical records are copied to their GP and this forms a record "from the cradle to the grave." Some data can be lost when patients move practices if a different computer system is used, although in the UK a process for transmitting

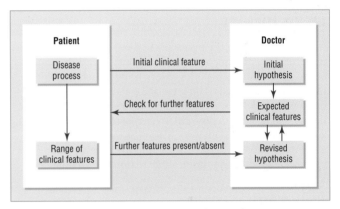

The hypothetico-deductive process used by skilled decision makers when assessing patients

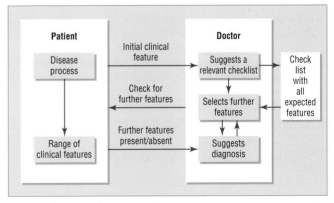

Inductive process using a checklist of symptoms. This way of assessing patients' problems is used by doctors who have less experience or experienced doctors who are dealing with an unfamiliar problem

records between GPs has been developed. In other countries patients are able to consult more than one primary care provider and a record held by the patient, such as a smart card, may be a more effective means of collecting the information needed to provide medical care safely. An alterative to smart cards might be subdermal devices that would allow access to data supplied by the patient anywhere in the world (see www.4verichip.com/verichip.htm).

Family history

Many causes of illness have intergenerational roots because of genetic or psychosocial factors. A doctor who knows that Mr Evans' mother had committed suicide when he was a child will be aware that both sets of factors may be operating in this case. On paper records, this information may not be identified easily on the summary sheet. Electronic records, however, present this information clearly as they contain information on past problems and current or active problems. Family doctors may have medical records of several members of extended families. The records can be accessed electronically, or the paper records can be read to identify patterns of illness that may not be apparent at the first consultation.

Drug history

In UK primary care, the repeat prescribing record is one of the most reliable components of the electronic record. As practices become increasingly paperless, more acute prescribing is captured electronically. The prescribing record can provide insights into the reason for the patient's attendance. Mr Evans has no diagnosis of depression in his record, but he did receive a tricyclic antidepressant twice before. Scanning the patient's treatment summary before calling him from the waiting room may alert the doctor to this possible reason for attendance.

Laboratory results

The slight macrocytosis and raised γ-glutamyltransferase levels detected after Mr Evan's visit to the practice a month ago alert Dr McKay to the possibility of an underlying alcohol problem. Mr Evans had been asked to come in again and the tests were repeated yesterday, and are now available on Dr McKay's computer to discuss with Mr Evans. Single results are often less informative than repeated values, which produce a discernible pattern. Some patients consult to obtain laboratory results. Results of tests sent out by mail are often delayed and patients appreciate the rapid access to results that laboratory links to practices allow. The need to interpret many results, taking into account a variety of factors, means that few results are sent directly to patients in the UK (in contrast to the United States). Decision support tools that annotate clinical, laboratory, or electrocardiogram reports with an interpretation may be helpful, and they are increasingly being used routinely.

Preconsultation screening

Dr McKay thinks that Mr Evans has psychological problems. This assessment is based on Dr McKay's knowledge of the patient and his family. This is confirmed when Mr Evans hands him the printed report from the hospital anxiety and depression rating scale, which he had completed on a computer in the waiting room. Preconsultation screening tools will probably become important features of family practice when their diagnostic and prognostic value is realised.

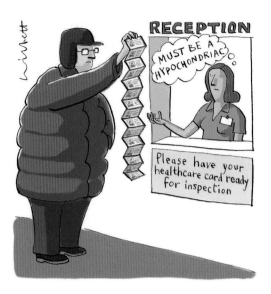

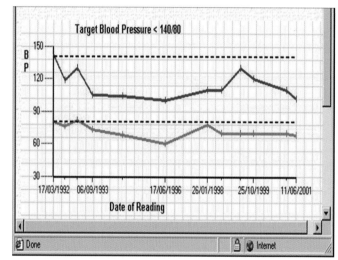

Cumulative recording of blood pressure

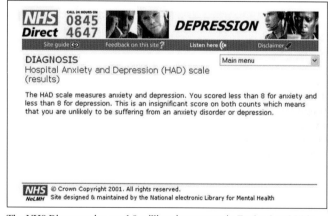

The NHS Direct service, used 8 million times a year in England and Wales, electronically delivers problem solving algorithms to assist triage nurses and patients to decide if a consultation is necessary. In the case of depression, a patient may believe that a GP is likely to offer drugs, and they may prefer to try non-pharmacological treatment

Direct patient data collection to replace follow-up consultations

Technological advances mean that temperature, pulse, blood pressure, peak flow rate, coagulation, blood, and urine chemistry can all be monitored at home and these data made available in graphical or tabular format during or instead of a consultation. Ambulatory blood pressure monitoring helps differentiate between a casual elevated blood pressure and sustained hypertension. Technology means that many of these data could be available continuously. Computer assisted interviews may also be used to obtain information before a follow-up visit to a doctor. A variety of health status measures with global and multidimensional scales can provide information to augment the clinical encounter.

Coding of clinical data

Text, images, sounds, and many other sources of data can be stored and retrieved by computers, but for computers to "understand" the data it must be put into a code. Until the onset of the information age coding and classification of data in any format was not considered an urgent task during consultations. Medical records have often been viewed mainly as aides memoire and secondarily as legal documents. To manage patients within an integrated health service it is becoming more important to communicate information from one setting in a digital format while retaining meaning when viewed in a different context. Although computerised text retains its meaning when communicating between humans, there are a variety of systems for coding and classification used to communicate meaning to computers. Two of the most widely used coding systems are Read (developed by Dr James Read and about 2000 other doctors), and SNOMED (Systematised Nomenclature of Medicine). The two systems are being combined into SNOMED-CT. Technically, these systems are multiaxial and hierarchical, but there are other classification systems with their own characteristics. Fortunately, most data can be interchanged from one to the other, albeit with loss of definition. The quality of coding, which varies between doctors, clinics, wards, and practices, will probably improve, driven by financial imperatives and facilitated by better functionality of the electronic record.

Using data from confidential sources

Family members may impart information about other members of their household to the GP, and by so doing, invite the doctor to act. In this case Mrs Evans had reported her husband's excessive alcohol consumption, his mood swings, and her fear of violence. Recording the allegation in his wife's notes is a straightforward and necessary step, as is making a record about advice given to her about her own safety, and a request that she ask Mr Evans to consult. Placing a record of this uncorroborated allegation in Mr Evans record, however, is more hazardous. Even referring to the suspicion when he does consult may cause marital difficulties if he exercises his rights under the data protection act 1998 to read his medical records.

> **In vulnerable, elderly patients, it may be particularly valuable to be able to measure temperature, pulse, blood pressure, peak flow rate, coagulation, blood, and urine chemistry at home and have these data made available for doctors**

Coding and classification

- Code—the numeric or alphabetic representation of data for the purpose of computer communication or processing
- Classification—a systematic arrangement of similar kinds of concepts such as diseases, on the basis of how they differ (for example, by aetiology)

Further reading

- Blau JN. How to take a history of head or facial pain. *BMJ* 1982;285:1249-51
- Schoenberg R, Safran C. Internet based repository of medical records that retains patient confidentiality. *BMJ* 2000;321:1199-1203
- Benson T. Why general practitioners use computers and hospital doctors do not—Part 1: incentives. *BMJ* 2002;325:1086-9
- Murff HJ, Gandhi TK, Karson AK, Mort EA, Poon EG, Wang SJ, et al. Primary care physician attitudes concerning follow-up of abnormal test results and ambulatory decision support systems. *Int J Med Inf* 2003;71:137-49
- Zigmond AS, Snaith RP. The Hospital Anxiety and Depression Scale. *Acta Psychiatr Scand* 1983;67:361-70
- Stewart AL, Greenfield S, Hays RD, Wells KB, Rogers WH, Berry SD, et al (1989). Functional status and well-being of patients with chronic conditions. *JAMA* 1989;262, 907-13
- www.bma.org.uk/ap.nsf/Content/accesshealthrecords (accessed 6 September 2005)

4 How decision support tools help define clinical problems

The patient, Mr Evans, presented with headaches and early morning wakening (dealt with in chapter 3) as the main reason for his consultation. This article, however, discusses how informatics resources can be used to consider issues other than the presenting problem. The Stott and Davies model of the consultation indicates that three other areas of the interaction should be considered.

- Management of continuing problems—The patient's diabetes may be contributing to the overall picture.
- Opportunistic health promotion—Ask screening questions about alcohol use and measure the patient's blood pressure.
- Modification of help seeking behaviours—Discuss issues relevant to self care and when to attend for health checks for established or potential problems.

Management of continuing problems

Awareness of problems

Sometimes doctors and patients are not aware of relevant problems. Issues that are apparent to one person may not be apparent to the other. In Mr Evans's case the diabetes is known to doctor and patient. The alcohol problem is, perhaps dimly, apparent to Mr Evans. The high blood pressure reading is something that only the doctor is aware of initially. Neither doctor nor patient is aware of the depression at the beginning of the consultation, but information conveyed before, or during, the consultation may alter that.

When a health professional realises that he or she is aware of an issue that the patient is not, the matter can be remedied. It is more difficult if the patient is aware of an issue that is relevant, but is unwilling to divulge it. Even more difficult is a situation where neither patient nor doctor is aware of a problem that may be relevant to the patient's problems (see Johari Window). Electronic prompts to bring up such hidden issues are being incorporated into clinical systems, and are increasingly effective.

Problems underlying depression

Depression is common and often associated with anxiety, cognitive impairment, and substance misuse.

It is important to detect alcohol misuse because failure to do so may mean that treatment for the presenting problem is ineffective. Several screening tools with different characteristics for various clinical settings are available. When the CAGE questionnaire is used on its own in primary care, a positive response to two or more items on it has a sensitivity of 93% and a specificity of 76%. Different questionnaire screening tests for alcohol misuse, such as the fast alcohol screening test (FAST), may detect problems at an early stage, when intervention may be more effective than later on. Other clues can help the doctor, including comments from family members and the nature of past consultations—for example, injuries that were only partially explained.

When the baseline probability of a condition and the odds ratio of a modifying factor are known, then the effect of any new information can be calculated by using Bayes' nomogram. Unfortunately, key items of information needed for such calculations are often unavailable. For the foreseeable future, interpreting the results of most investigations still relies heavily

Mr Evans is a 49 year old, recently unemployed, pharmaceutical company representative who has presented with low mood, poor appetite, and sleep disturbance. He drinks two bottles of whisky per week, but he does not volunteer this information initially. He has type 2 diabetes. A blood pressure check shows 178/114 mm Hg, and Mr Evans is asked to return to the practice nurse for follow-up

Management of presenting problems	Modification of help seeking behaviours
Management of continuing problems	Opportunistic health promotion

Exceptional potential in each consultation. Adapted from Stott NCH, Davies RH. *J Roy Coll Gen Pract* 1979;29:201-5

	Known to patient	Not known to patient
Known to clinician	Open	Blind
Not known to clinician	Hidden	Unknown

The Johari Window shows situations where one or both individuals in the consultation may not be aware of all the relevant information

Baseline probability	Odds ratio	Post-exposure probability
0.01		0.99
0.02		0.98
0.03	1000	0.97
0.05	500	0.95
0.07		0.93
0.1	100	0.9
	50	
0.2		0.8
0.3	10	0.7
0.4	5	0.6
0.5	1	0.5
0.6	0.5	0.4
0.7		0.3
0.8	0.1	0.2
	0.05	
0.9	0.01	0.1
0.01	0.005	0.07
0.93		0.05
0.95	0.001	0.03
0.97		0.02
0.99		0.01

When estimates of the odds ratio and baseline probability are known, Bayes' nomogram can be used to calculate post-exposure probability

on (according to Feinstein) "the judgements of thoughtful people who are familiar with the total realities of human ailments."

Apart from depression, there are other situations in which harmful alcohol use may be important, and an electronic alert may be useful in a consultation. Although it is not the main reason for consulting, Mr Evans also has type 2 diabetes and today's consultation is an opportunity to deliver proactive care.

Problems complicating diabetes

The microvascular and macrovascular complications of type 2 diabetes need to be monitored regularly. Guidelines are incorporated into local clinical governance structures to ensure that all necessary care is given to patients. Organisations are responsible for providing different elements of the care recorded in electronic patient records. Integrated services (such as health maintenance organisations or the managed clinical network) share responsibilities, using electronic health records across primary, secondary, and tertiary care.

Mr Evans's only abnormal physical test result is a blood pressure of 178/114 mm Hg. The raised blood pressure is potentially important, and the practice's decision support software gives advice on what to do next. Most of the advice on checking for secondary causes of hypertension (such as excessive alcohol ingestion and end organ damage) is familiar to the doctor, as is the advice to repeat the examination on several occasions before starting treatment. Grade 1 evidence from meta-analyses or large randomised controlled trials may be available for straightforward clinical problems (for example, starting antihypertensive drugs), but this is not always the case.

Clinical decision support tools are being refined to provide the information that clinicians require without overloading them with unnecessary data. This is difficult as the amount of information needed and the sources from which information is obtained varies.

Guidelines

Field and Lohr describe clinical practice guidelines as "systematically developed statements to assist practitioners and patient decisions about appropriate health care for specific circumstances." One role of guidelines is to ensure that all relevant issues are dealt with during clinical encounters. Individual guideline organisations have their own websites and other organisations, such as the Turning Research into Practice (TRIP) database, integrate several guideline sources and other evidence based resources.

Computerised guidelines provide evidence based recommendations for, and can automatically generate recommendations about, the screening, diagnostic, or therapeutic activities that are suggested for a specific patient. The advantages of computerised guidelines over written guidelines are that they:
- Provide readily accessible references and allow access to knowledge in guidelines that have been selected for use in a specific clinical context
- Show errors or anachronisms in the content of a guideline
- Often improve the clarity of a guideline
- Can be tailored to a patient's clinical state
- Propose timely decision support that is specific for the patient
- Send reminders.

Knowledge from unfamiliar sources

In the post-genomic world, clinicians will have to integrate their understanding of patients' phenotype with new information

Highest scoring diabetes indicators in UK GP Quality and Outcomes Framework 2004*

Indicator	Points	Maximum threshold
Records		
Practice can produce a register of all patients with diabetes mellitus	6	
Ongoing management		
Percentage of patients with diabetes in whom the last HbA1c is 7.4 or less (or equivalent test/reference range depending on local laboratory) in past 15 months	16	50%
Percentage of patients with diabetes in whom the last HbA1c is 10 or less (or equivalent test or reference range depending on local laboratory) in past 15 months	11	85%
Percentage of patients with diabetes who have a record of retinal screening in the previous 15 months	5	90%
Percentage of patients with diabetes in whom the last blood pressure is 145/85 mm Hg or less	17	55%
Percentage of patients with diabetes whose last measured total cholesterol within previous 15 months is 5 or less	6	60%

*In total, 1050 quality points are available, of which 550 points are for clinical targets. The most important areas are coronary heart disease, hypertension, and diabetes, which account for 325 (59%) of the 550 points for clinical indicators

---

Revised grading system for recommendations in evidence based guidelines*

Levels of evidence
1++ High quality meta-analyses, systematic reviews of RCTs, or RCTs with a very low risk of bias
1+ Well conducted meta-analyses, systematic reviews of RCTs, or RCTs with a low risk of bias
1– Meta-analyses, systematic reviews or RCTs, or RCTs with a high risk of bias
2++ High quality systematic reviews of case-control or cohort studies *or* high quality case-control or cohort studies with a very low risk of confounding, bias, or chance and a high probability that the relationship is causal
2+ Well conducted case-control or cohort studies with a low risk of confounding, bias, or chance and a moderate probability that the relationship is causal
2– Case-control or cohort studies with a high risk of confounding, bias, or chance and a significant risk that the relationship is not causal
3 Non-analytic studies—for example, case reports, case series
4 Expert opinion

Grades of recommendations
A At least one meta-analysis, systematic review, or RCT rated as 1++ and directly applicable to the target population *or*
A systematic review of RCTs or a body of evidence consisting principally of studies rated as 1+ directly applicable to the target population and demonstrating overall consistency of results
B A body of evidence including studies rated as 2++ directly applicable to the target population and demonstrating overall consistency of results *or*
Extrapolated evidence from studies rated as 1++ or 1+
C A body of evidence including studies rated as 2+ directly applicable to the target population and demonstrating overall consistency of results *or*
Extrapolated evidence from studies rated as 2++
D Evidence level 3 or 4 *or*
Extrapolated evidence from studies rated as 2+

*Guidelines of the Scottish Intercollegiate Guidelines Network Grading Review Group. RCT = randomised controlled trial

from genomics, proteomics, and metabonomics. These new modes of inquiry about patients' underlying genetic status help to explain older, empirical observations. For example, the relative ineffectiveness of aspirin in preventing thromboembolic disorders in 25% of the population may be caused by several common gene variants that affect platelet glycoprotein function. The challenge to clinicians is to integrate this new knowledge into their diagnostic and therapeutic approaches during consultations.

Modifying help seeking behaviours

Some patients with long term health problems do not attend review appointments. This is a particular problem when the individual has multiple comorbidities. A patient with depression may not think it is worthwhile spending scarce health service resources on themselves because they have low self esteem, which is often associated with depression. Electronic patient records summarise health problems and, potentially, prompt when reviews have not been undertaken. Some services, like review of the patient's self monitoring, can be provided immediately. Others, such as retinopathy screening, may have to be scheduled for another date and place. An electronic health record shared between colleagues in different professions and parts of the health services makes scheduling easier.

Electronic clinical information systems

The principal function of electronic clinical information systems is to facilitate patient care. This involves identifying, classifying, understanding, and resolving problems to the satisfaction of the patients. Clinical records are also required to recall observations, to inform others, to instruct students, to gain knowledge, to monitor performance, and to justify intervention. Electronic clinical information systems are becoming integral components of healthcare services, and in many industrialised countries they are replacing the established paper based system of records. Combining the electronic patient records of different organisations creates a single electronic health record. The challenge for many health services is to provide "cradle to grave" information. Effective integration of records depends on establishing a workable unique patient identification system such as the community health index.

Summary

Individuals in most industrial societies who are, or believe themselves to be, ill can turn to a variety of sources of advice other than health professionals. However, these sources will probably only help with the problems that a person deals with that day. A doctor is often needed to provide additional information, and to interpret and individualise advice for all the problems brought to the consultation by the patient, not just the presenting problem.

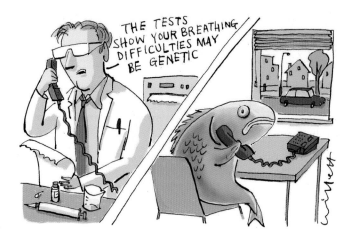

Definitions
- Electronic patient record—Records the periodic care provided mainly by one institution. Typically, this information will relate to the health care given to a patient by an acute hospital
- Electronic health record—A longitudinal record of patients' health and health care: from cradle to grave. It combines the information about patient contacts with primary health care as well as subsets of information associated with the outcomes of periodic care held in the electronic patient record

Further reading
- Brief description of Johari Window on practice: www.freemaninstitute.com/johari.htm
- Bodenheimer T, Grumbach K. Electronic technology: a spark to revitalize primary care? *JAMA.* 2003;290:259-64
- McCusker, MT, Basquille J, Khwaja M, Murray-Lyon IM, Catalan J. Hazardous and harmful drinking: a comparison of the AUDIT and CAGE screening questionnaires. *Quart J Med* 2002;95:591-5
- Page J, Attia J. Using Bayes' nomogram to help interpret odds ratios. *Evidence Based Med* 2003;8:132-4
- Feinstein AR. The need for humanised science in evaluating medication. *Lancet* 1972;297:421-3
- Field MJ, Lohr KN, eds. *Guidelines for clinical practice: from development to use.* Washington DC: National Academy Press, 1992
- TRIP database: www.tripdatabase.com
- Bray PF. Platelet glycoprotein polymorphisms as risk factors for thrombosis *Curr Opin Haematol* 2000;7:284-9
- Smith R. The future of healthcare systems. *BMJ* 1997;314:1495-6
- Wyatt JC. *Clinical knowledge and practice in the information age: a handbook for health professionals.* London: Royal Society of Medicine Press, 2001
- Community Health Index (CHI) in Scotland. www.show.scot.nhs.uk/ehealth/

5 How computers can help to share understanding with patients

In chapter 2 Ms Patel found a lot of material on the internet and spoke to family members about their health and the causes of death of some family members. Ms Patel discussed this information with her general practitioner (GP), who then referred Ms Patel to a clinical genetics centre. The genetics clinic team converted Ms Patel's understanding of the situation into a genogram using Risk Assessment in Genetics software (RAGs).

A cancer registry was used to find the cause of death of Ms Patel's older sister because she had died overseas. By integrating multiple sources of information the genetics clinic team could advise Ms Patel that her lifetime risk of developing breast cancer was about 30%, and that she would probably benefit from further investigation. If Ms Patel was investigated and shown to carry the BRCA1 gene, the risk estimate for Ms Patel's nieces would be higher.

Before doctors introduce information to patients they should determine the way in which patients want to look for information, discover their level of knowledge on the subject, elicit any specific concerns they have, and find out the information that they need. Interactive health communication applications, such as decision support tools and websites, give doctors and patients additional ways to share understanding of patients' reasons for consulting, and they can then work together to solve patients' problems. The benefits to patients of using interactive health communication applications include a better understanding of their health problems, reduced uncertainty, and the feeling that they are getting better support from their carers.

Many of these tools are new and unfamiliar to patients and doctors. The best way to use them to achieve better outcomes for patients during the time available in consultations remains to be established. Research indicates that patients would like to be directed to a high quality interactive health communication application at diagnosis, and at any decision point thereafter (E Murray, personal communication, 2004).

Ms Amulya Patel is a 48 year old accountant whose mother and possibly two sisters have had breast cancer. Because of her family history, clinical examination and mammography were undertaken. Mammography indicated an area of microcalcification in the upper outer quadrant of her left breast

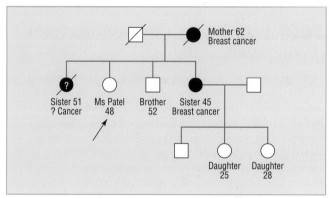

A patient's view of risk, presented as a three generation genogram

Access to images, audio, and animation

The mammogram, like other clinical images, is available as hard copy or as an archived picture delivered to the desktop of any clinician authorised to view it. The image may be presented with extra material to help explain the nature of the problem. Archived images are more likely to be available than a film, and serial display of archived copies allows comparison.

Many patients like explanation in the form of a diagram or in simple, often anatomical, terms. Some patients, however, prefer more detailed descriptions (for example, pathological explanations) of what is happening to their body. This information can be provided by clinicians on their computer screens, using digitised slide libraries, CD Roms, or material on websites.

Multimedia information retrieval

Large documents can be stored and transferred rapidly over electronic and optical fibre networks. These documents may include pictures, sound, video, or computer programs, such as

---

Patient information

Patients need information to
- Understand what is wrong
- Gain a realistic idea of prognosis
- Make the most of consultations
- Understand the processes and likely outcomes of tests and treatment
- Help in self care
- Learn about available services and sources of help
- Provide reassurance and help
- Help others understand
- Legitimise their concerns and the need to seek help
- Learn how to prevent further illness
- Identify further information and self help groups
- Identify the best healthcare providers

---

simulators. Textbooks, journal articles, clinical guidelines, image libraries, and material designed for patient education are increasingly becoming available electronically. Discussing individual electronic health records and relevant reference material with patients is preferable to discussing general information about their problem. If Ms Patel and her surgeon are discussing whether she may need a lumpectomy or a simple mastectomy, then the ability to view a relevant image and brief text making the comparison will probably be more effective than a comprehensive treatise on all the possible procedures.

Risk prediction tools

During the discussion of a potentially serious problem like breast cancer, the issue of prognosis will probably arise. Until recently prognostication has been largely implicit, and it was based on the clinical experience of similar patients with the same kind of problems and comorbidities. In a few cases (such as head injury or seriously ill patients in the intensive care unit) accurate, well calibrated clinical prediction rules like the Glasgow coma scale are available. Databases that contain information about patients with known characteristics are being developed, and this information is available across a range of specialties to augment clinicians' experience with the type of problem they are dealing with.

Problems with information retrieval during consultations

Although much information is at hand, it is often difficult to find the most clinically relevant items. Studies measuring the use of information resources during consultations showed individual clinicians accessed the resources only a few times a month. To encourage clinicians to make more use of these information resources, other approaches to information retrieval during the encounter are being studied.

● Email or telephone access to a human searcher—An example is the ATTRACT question answering service for clinicians working in Wales

● Human annotation—This approach uses links between relevant documents and a selected set of common queries that are manually assigned by a peer group (for example, by all the breast surgeons in Scotland or a group of radiologists in New England) for mutual reference

● Case based reasoning—A generic approach to problem solving developed by researchers in the field of artificial intelligence. Problems are solved by adapting new solutions to similar problems that have already been solved

● Automatic query construction—Information from an electronic medical record is used to construct the query, partially or fully. Approaches include interactive user selection of terms, automatic recognition of MeSH index terms in the text of medical records, and developing generic queries that can be filled in with terms from the record

● Search by navigation—In this approach it is possible to search for information by traversing links between information items rather than constructing a query. Fixed links may be organised in a hierarchical menu or as hypertext. Links may also be created dynamically to reflect the changing needs of the user.

Computers in a consultation

The computer screen requires more attention than notes on paper, and clinicians spend less time interacting with the patient

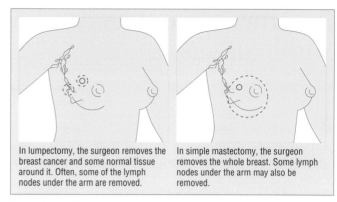

In lumpectomy, the surgeon removes the breast cancer and some normal tissue around it. Often, some of the lymph nodes under the arm are removed.

In simple mastectomy, the surgeon removes the whole breast. Some lymph nodes under the arm may also be removed.

Comparison of lumpectomy and mastectomy—simple diagrams with brief text can be effective in consultations. Adapted from http://medem.com/medlb/article_detaillb.cfm?article_ID=ZZZSOTZD38C&sub_cat=57

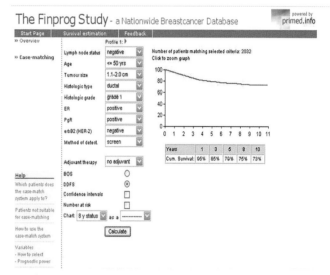

The Finprog study uses data on a large number of patients with breast cancer to allow an individualised prediction of survival for a new patient by matching their disease profile to that of other patients whose outcomes are known. From the website www.finprog.org

Problems with real time searches during consultations

● Time is spent composing and typing queries for each resource

● Indexing vocabularies are designed by and for librarians and are inconsistent and non-intuitive for clinicians

● Search programs and their displays are designed for research and educational purposes, not for use at the point of care

● No provision for system initiative; that is, clinicians can only find what they choose to look for. A relevant document may exist in the clinical trials resource, but if the doctor thinks that finding a clinical trial is unlikely, then that resource will not be searched

● Although many clinical situations occur often, it is difficult to reuse or share retrieval success

● Managing and updating the information resources is an extra responsibility for the doctor when they use information resources during consultations. Despite this, doctors who use computers during their consultations are viewed favourably by patients. Research is needed to investigate how additional electronic information resources can be integrated into the consultation, given that a patient centred consultation style is desirable.

After the consultation

It may be difficult, or impossible, to share understanding of all important issues with a patient during the limited time available in many clinical environments. Difficult, embarrassing, or additional questions may occur to the patient after leaving the clinic. Written material (preprinted or produced during the consultation), audiotapes of the consultation, or an email with relevant website links for the patient may provide another chance for them or their carers to revisit the issues or extend a line of inquiry that was partially dealt with in the consultation.

Summary

One of the most attractive features of integrating multimedia information into the consultation is that the process educates and empowers patient and doctor. Jointly, they retain control over the conduct and conclusions of the encounter. In particular, bringing information to the point of care allows the patient to participate in decision making, and encourages them to learn from the doctor's expertise in interpreting and critically appraising information, rather than depending on the doctor's memory and powers of recall.

At present sources of relevant, well prepared, evidence based material are insufficient. Systematic reviews and other assessments of health technology could be amended to include sections presenting information for patients on the choices of treatment that they have, with input from relevant patient groups. Guidance from NICE (the National Institute for Health and Clinical Excellence) always includes a detailed information leaflet, but this can only be as evidence based as the available research allows. Some patients will prefer to discuss their problems during consultations with a doctor they trust, but audiovisual aids can help that process during and after the consultation.

Further reading

- Emery J, Walton R, Coulson A, Glasspool D, Ziebland S, Fox J. A qualitative evaluation of computer support for recording and interpreting family histories of breast and ovarian cancer in primary care (RAGs) using simulated cases. *BMJ* 1999;319:32-6
- Murray E, Burns J, See-Tai S, Lai R, Nazareth I. Interactive Health Communication Applications for people with chronic disease. *Cochrane Database Syst Rev* 2004;(4):CD4274
- Jones R, Pearson J, McGregor S, Cawsey AJ, Barret A, Craig N, et al. Randomised trial of personalised computer based information for cancer patients. *BMJ* 1999;319:1241-7
- Schmidt H.G. Norman GR, Boshuizen HPA. A cognitive perspective on medical expertise: theory and implications. *Academic medicine* 1990;65:611-21
- Jennett B, Teasdale G, Braakman R, Minderhoud J, Knill-Jones R. Predicting outcome in ndividual patients after severe head injury. *Lancet* 1976;1:1031-4
- Hersh WR, Hickam DH. How well do physicians use electronic information retrieval systems? A framework for investigation and systematic review. *JAMA* 1998;280:1347-52
- Brassey J, Elwyn G, Price C, Kinnersley P. Just in time information for clinicians: a questionnaire evaluation of the ATTRACT project. *BMJ* 2001;322:529-30
- Ridsdale L, Hudd S. Computers in the consultation: the patient's view. *Br J Gen Pract* 1994;44:367-9
- Dickinson D, Raynor DKT. Ask the patients—they may want to know more than you think. *BMJ* 2003;327:861
- Lundin J, Lundin M, Isola J, Joensuu H. A web-based system for individualised survival estimation in breast cancer. *BMJ* 2003;326:29

6   How informatics tools help deal with patients' problems

During the everyday general practice consultation described in the box opposite, the common and rare collide. A problem that may have been a routine matter becomes one of enormous importance to the doctor and the patient. At least seven problems should be dealt with during the consultation. This article, which follows on from the initial contact between Dr McKay and Ms Smith described in chapter 1, explains how a range of solutions may be presented to doctors during the consultation to augment their decision making processes.

Presenting problems

Ms Smith came to see her GP because of tiredness and muscle cramps, and these problems need to be considered in detail. Potential solutions should be discussed with Ms Smith in a way that she can understand.

The patient's history indicated that, among other things, her pulse should be taken and her blood pressure measured. The abnormal physical findings recorded in the electronic notes were pallor and a blood pressure of 178/114 mm Hg. The raised blood pressure was a potentially important new finding, and the practice's decision support software gave advice on what to do next. Most of the advice on checking for secondary causes of hypertension and end organ damage was familiar to Dr McKay, as was the recommendation on PRODIGY (Prescribing RatiOnally with Decision Support) to repeat the examination on several occasions before starting treatment.

The rest of this article describes Ms Smith's return visit, when several blood pressure recordings and routine biochemistry test results were available to Dr McKay. Clinical decision support tools are being refined to provide the knowledge that doctors need without overloading them with unnecessary advice. This goal may be difficult to achieve because the amount of information needed varies between health professionals and clinical situations.

Investigation

Four hours after the practice nurse had sent the patient's blood for testing, the results arrived by email. Ms Smith's result had been flagged red, and so Dr McKay opened up the details and saw that she had substantial renal impairment, hyperkalaemia, and hypercalcaemia of sufficient severity to explain her presenting symptoms. Having laboratory test results available on the same day the tests are done can reduce delays in starting treatment. An urgent phone call or email from the laboratory may be preferred for extremely abnormal results, like a serum potassium 6.7 mmol/l.

Ambulatory blood pressure readings can be made available through telemetry or at the patient's next visit to determine whether there is a sustained rise in blood pressure. An increasing number of biometric sensing devices can provide information to help with the decision making process.

> **Ms Smith is a 58 year old florist with a 15 year history of renal impairment caused by childhood pyelonephritis. She has tiredness and muscle cramps. She consulted her general practitioner (GP), Dr McKay, three days ago. Dr McKay noted Ms Smith's blood pressure was 178/114 mm Hg, and she asked her to visit the practice nurse (who could repeat Ms Smith's blood pressure test) to check her urinalysis and send off blood for laboratory tests. The results of the blood tests show serum potassium 5.2 mmol/l, serum calcium 2.8 mmol/l with albumin 38 g/l, and creatinine 567 µmol/l**

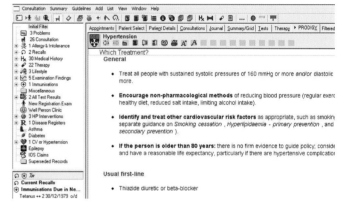

Decision support for hypertension

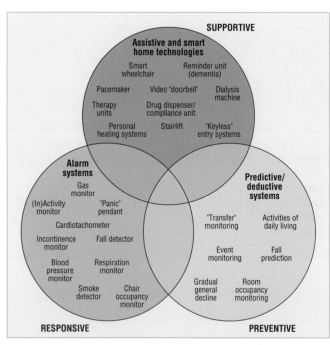

A wide range of sensing devices are available and can be broadly categorised

Referral

At the next visit Dr McKay tells Ms Smith that she should start treatment for hypertension and hypercalcaemia. Dr McKay also says that Ms Smith should be referred to a renal physician, Dr Jones, and a community dietitian for further assessment. Ms Smith agrees, and Dr McKay telephones the hospital to discuss these matters during the consultation. Dr McKay then uses an electronic referral form on the hospital outpatient booking website to provide the information required by colleagues at the local hospital. In some contexts, this final task can be done using an electronic booking programme. Health maintenance organisations in the United States, which provide integrated primary and secondary care, book appointments electronically, and the ability to do this is a priority in the United Kingdom. Booking appointments electronically in more complex referral settings is difficult. The problem is not a technical one—rather, political and workflow difficulties make transfer of meaningful data between different parts of a health service hard to achieve.

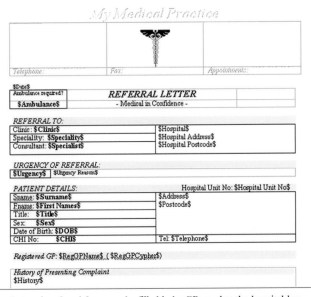

An electronic referral form can be filled in by GPs so that the hospital has all the necessary details of the patient

"Just in time" learning

Dr McKay had missed an issue of the *BMJ* in which it was reported that blood pressures taken during consultations are often inaccurate. However, the article in question had loaded automatically into the *Clinical Evidence* folders of the file storage on her Palmtop computer. Alternatively, the article could be held on a laptop computer, mobile phone, or in a secure personal web file to allow remote access.

This new knowledge was available to Dr McKay during the first consultation, and she asked the practice nurse to arrange ambulatory blood pressure testing. This is an example of a "push technology," which makes information available when and where it is needed—just in time. When an interest is registered in clinical topics relevant to a practice, selected and relevant information can be sent to the practice by email, or mobile phone text messages or downloads, at daily or weekly intervals, or less often. Most doctors, whether in hospital or the community, are rarely in one place for long. The information systems they use to support their work need to be as mobile as they are. Technological advances allow doctors to access data and knowledge when connected to a fixed source like a CD Rom of their favourite book or by wireless connection to the internet.

Reasons for using handheld computers at the point of care in the United States in 2003

- To access drug information—67%
- To access clinical decision support—22%
- To prescribe drugs—13%
- To access medical records—4%
- To view laboratory results—3%

High quality information portals for patients

- www.nhsdirect.nhs.uk
- www.patient.co.uk
- www.omni.ac.uk
- www.noah-health.org/en/rights

See also: Potts HWW; Wyatt JC. Survey of doctors' experience of patients using the internet. *J Med Internet Res* 2002. www.jmir.org/2002/1/e5/

Accessing information after the consultation

At the end of the consultation Dr McKay emails Ms Smith the address of a good website containing information aimed at patients so that she can access it from home, a public library, or an internet cafe. The availability of high quality resources for patients mitigates potentially alarming messages on less scrupulous websites that may, for example, say that high blood pressure is often caused by mercury poisoning from dental fillings.

Most GPs accept that patient education is an important consultation task. They may be sceptical about whether patients take their advice on smoking and exercise, but doctors continue to tailor advice to patients because specific information does improve knowledge and reduces any conflict that might arise during decision making. Educating patients need not be limited by short consultation times.

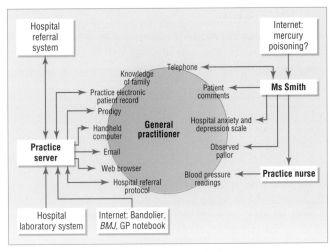

Information used during and around the consultation

Summary

This episode of care illustrates many of the features of medicine in the information age. People in industrial societies who are, or believe themselves to be, ill can turn to a variety of sources of advice other than health professionals. In most cases these resources, personal knowledge, and advice from family and friends will be enough for people to resolve their health problems. In other cases, the information they obtain will be insufficient or misleading. A primary care clinician is often needed to provide additional information, interpret it, and individualise advice for each of the problems brought to the consultation by the patient. A few patients may seem reluctant to seek information or participate in decisions about treatment options. They prefer being told what to do, but even these patients usually appreciate a paper leaflet or website address that they can give to family or friends who are more enquiring.

In this example, some of the problems that had to be dealt with included Ms Smith's presenting problems (tiredness and muscle cramps); opportunistic health promotion (screening for anxiety and depression), managing ongoing problems (metabolic upset and hypertension caused by chronic pyelonephritis), and modifying help seeking behaviours (easing the patient's uncertainty over electronic information sources).

Dr McKay had to decide on and undertake seven actions during this consultation.
- Explaining the cause of the patient's symptoms and available treatments in a way that Ms Smith could understand
- Assuaging the patient's anxiety that she may have mercury poisoning
- Starting treatment for hypertension with a thiazide
- Starting treatment for hypercalcaemia with bisphosphonates
- Referring Ms Smith to a consultant nephrologist
- Referring Ms Smith to a community dietitian
- Advising the patient on use of internet resources to obtain more information

Fortunately, clinicians in primary care teams no longer need to rely on memories of lectures or their old medical textbooks. Better informed patients, medical records that inform and teach, and electronic sources of reliable, well presented information make it easier to make informed decisions on problems presented in primary care. Informatics tools are generally less helpful in more complex situations, in which there may be uncertainty about the outcomes of interventions or no professional consensus on the value of the outcomes that are achievable.

Better decisions in primary care should lead to more appropriate referrals to secondary care and a more efficient health service. Research on the information needs of primary care clinicians is informing the development of information services. Educational research is starting to show how to meet those educational needs most effectively and in a manner congruent with professional revalidation.

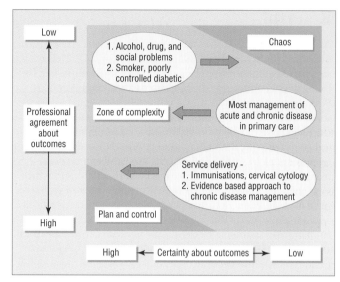

Certainty and professional agreement on clinical decision making. Adapted from Hassey A. Complexity and the clinical encounter. In Sweeney K, Griffiths F (eds). *Complexity and healthcare: and introduction* Oxford: Radcliffe Medical Press, 2002

Further reading

- Poon EG, Wang SJ, Gandhi TK, Bates DW, Kuperman GJ. Design and implementation of a comprehensive outpatient Results Manager. *J Biomed Inform* 2003;36:80-91
- Choose and book website: www.chooseandbook.nhs.uk/ (accessed 6 Oct 2005)
- Little P, Barnett J, Barnsley L, Marjoram J, Fitzgerald-Barron A, Mant D. Comparison of agreement between different measures of blood pressure in primary care and daytime ambulatory blood pressure. *BMJ* 2002;325:254
- Smith R. The future of health care systems. *BMJ* 1997;314:1495-6
- Wyatt JC. *Clinical knowledge and practice in the information age: a handbook for health professionals.* London: Royal Society of Medicine Press, 2001
- Ely JW, Osheroff JA, Ebell MH, Chambliss ML, Vinson DC, Stevermer JJ, Pifer EA. Obstacles to answering doctors' questions about patient care with evidence: qualitative study. *BMJ* 2002;324:71
- Peck C, McCall M, McLaren B, Rotem T. Continuing medical education and continuing professional development: international comparisons. *BMJ* 2000;320:432-5

7 How computers help make efficient use of consultations

Efficient consultations deal with patients' problems promptly and effectively while taking into account other relevant circumstances. Sometimes the relevant circumstance is another health problem in the patient or their family, or it could be an issue affecting society at large, such as resource constraints. The immediate role of the team caring for Patrick Murphy (see box opposite) is to deal with his severe asthma.

To do so the team needs information on the current problem, which is quickly obtained from Patrick's mother (who accompanied him in the ambulance) and background details from her or from his medical records. They also need to assess Patrick's physical status using clinical examination and other diagnostic methods. The information obtained enables the clinicians caring for Patrick to take the most effective management steps. In the longer term, data from the consultation may be used to redesign the service locally, or at the level of the health system. This article shows how informatics tools can make it easier to record important data, and that this processing can produce useful information for a low cost.

Most doctors focus on assessing the patient and carrying out immediate management steps. Some clinicians see the recording of what happened and why as a necessary evil to be done in the minimum time, with the least effort. Legal responsibilities ensure that most encounters are recorded, but the quality of data is often constrained, partly because so much data are required.

Data to be recorded for acute medical admissions

- Patient's registered general practice details
- Admission details (administrative)
- Reason for clinical encounter
- Presenting problem
- History of presenting problem
- Current diagnoses, problems
- Drugs, allergies, and diets
- Past illnesses, procedures, and investigations
- Social circumstances
- Functional state
- Family history
- Systems review
- Examination results
- Results of investigations
- Overall assessment and problem list
- Management plan
- Intended outcomes
- Information given to patient and carers

Write once, read many

Other tasks in the emergency consultation include gathering and recording information that may be useful to Patrick or other patients in the future. Paper or electronic records, or other information tools, may make it easier to record items of data that can be aggregated and analysed after the event. The data can improve efficiency when they are entered into clinical records and made available to other members of the clinical team. Wireless networks allow data to be transmitted to and from handheld computers, laptops, or desktop computers. This

> **Patrick Murphy is a 6 year old boy who has been brought to the accident and emergency department with status asthmaticus. He is cyanosed with a poor respiratory effort**

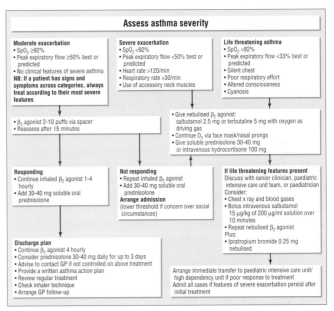

Acute asthma management flow chart for children >5 years in accident and emergency department. Adapted from Scottish Intercollegiate Guidelines Network, guideline 63 (www.sign.ac.uk/guidelines/fulltext/63/index.html)

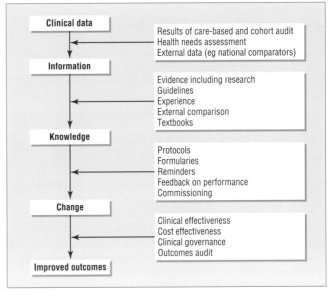

Turning clinical data into improved patient outcomes

19

enables data to be shared early. An improved standard of record keeping probably means better data in the electronic patient record, which increases knowledge about the range of problems seen in clinical practice. This new knowledge informs decisions made at several levels, and contributes to better outcomes for patients.

Structured recording of data

Although modern computers have massive processing and storage capacity, data needs to be recorded in code to be "understood" by computers. The computer processes and analyses the data to add meaning. Free text notes are too difficult for computers to process so that clinicians and policymakers can carry out analyses on them.

Although there are many coding and classification systems, according to Gardner, one system aims to "create a new world standard for computerising medical terminology." It is called the systematised nomenclature of medicine and clinical terms (SNOMED-CT) system. This coding system will be used in the NHS. It is a detailed, coded classification of medical terms and concepts, and has more than 150 000 terms and codes that are organised into 11 linked, hierarchical modules. Doctors will not see, and do not have to remember, all these codes. They use the interface provided by their clinical system, which is intuitive and carries out all the necessary translation to and from English.

To realise all potential efficiencies, the electronic record must comply with several requirements. The variables to be collected and their format may be agreed at different levels: hospital, region, organisation, or country. The electronic records should also be shared appropriately among different organisational units using standard communications procedures, and they must be subject to security and confidentiality protocols. Computer systems designed with sharing in mind are called "open." They can run programs that connect with systems of the same type, and can accept programs or connections from other sources.

Rapid decisions and the human brain

In Patrick Murphy's case, effective use of consultation data may not require a computer. Most clinical decision making is done faster than current computer technologies can manage.

Clinical prediction rules

A clinical prediction rule, sometimes called a clinical decision rule, is a method that quantifies the individual contributions made by various components of the history, examination, and basic laboratory results towards the diagnosis, prognosis, or likely response to treatment in a specific patient. Clinical prediction rules increase the accuracy of clinicians' diagnostic and prognostic assessments. They have been developed to help diagnose and manage patients with a wide range of diseases and in different settings. They reduce the uncertainty inherent in medical practice by defining how to use clinical findings to make predictions.

Every rule should assist the doctor in making a decision, and each one is based on factors drawn from a patient's history, physical examination, or diagnostic tests. The Ottawa ankle rule is often used. The Ottawa Health Research Institute keeps an inventory of clinical prediction rules. In August 2004 it recorded 523 prediction rules, 337 of which were validated using Cochrane methods.

Classification, coding, and nomenclature

- Classification is a method for systematically grouping something—for example, diseases. In most classifications, classes are designated by codes, which allow aspects of the things to be captured (a systematic arrangement of similar entities on the basis of certain characteristics)
- A code is usually a unique numeric or alphabetic representation of items in a classification
- Nomenclature is a system of naming used in a branch of knowledge. Medical nomenclature attempts to standardise the names used for patient findings, diseases, interventions, and outcomes

Secondary uses of data captured during consultations

- Reminders and decision support
- Communication of clinical data between healthcare workers—for example, discharge summaries, referrals, ordering, and requests
- Identifying and monitoring the health needs of a population
- Reducing bureaucracy while managing and funding care delivery
- Enabling reporting of externally specified health statistics—for example, for infection control
- Effective and efficient resource allocation and healthcare management
- Research
- Education
- Local clinical audit and governance

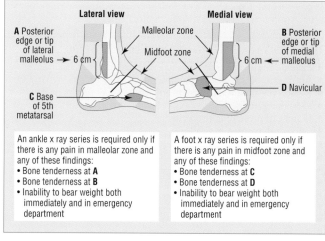

Ottawa ankle rules for use of radiography in acute ankle injuries. Adapted from Stiell IG, et al. *JAMA* 1994;271:827-32

Factors predicting a future risk of developing near-fatal or fatal asthma

- Socioeconomic deprivation
- Previous near fatal asthma—for example, previous ventilation or respiratory acidosis
- Previous admission for asthma, especially if in past year
- Requiring three or more classes of asthma medication
- Overuse of β_2 agonist
- Repeated attendance at accident and emergency department for asthma care, especially if in past year
- Brittle asthma
- Poor adherence to drug regimen

After decisions about how to manage a clinical problem have been made, admissions that are potentially avoidable should be considered. Using data to stratify the risk of recurrence may enable doctors to vary the level of follow-up and to tailor treatment depending on the risk—for example, the risk of Patrick's asthma recurring.

Establishing trust

An effective consultation instils trust and develops the relationship between doctor and patient. In Patrick's case, his family will probably consider returning to the team who dealt with his problems on this occasion for further care. When a patient sees the same doctor over time in a general practice surgery or outpatient clinic, it makes the consultation more efficient for both parties. The patient's story need not be repeated, and clinical examinations provide data that are comparable. When personal continuity of care is not possible, the electronic patient record provides some organisational continuity. Complete and accurate recording of data by clinicians becomes more important when a different member of the healthcare team needs to know what information is already known, or deduced, about the patient.

Efficient use of consultation time

The time available during consultations is often constrained, and doctors may need to select the most important problems to deal with. In a case like Patrick's, this is simple: the severity of his physical disease means that his acute respiratory problem must be managed. On a later occasion (for example, at the next outpatient visit) discussing parental smoking or pets in the house may be the best use of time. Looking over the patient's records before a consultation may alert the doctor to opportunities for efficient use of time. Patients often forget much of what is said during a consultation, and giving them an audio recording of consultations is an easy and cheap way for patients to listen to the advice provided after their visit is over. Providing patients with a written leaflet or advice about a self help organisation with materials on its website is also useful.

Summary

The strengths of human thought processes may be complemented by the strengths of electronic tools. The initial costs of developing and implementing new information systems may be high, but the costs thereafter can be lower than the non-electronic source that is being replaced. In 2003, American policymakers said that $120 billion a year could be saved by using information systems. Well designed, new, informatics tools typically improve effectiveness by 10-15%. Lower costs and better outcomes mean that informatics tools are moving from an era of hype to one in which real benefits are seen.

Continuity of care*

For patients and their families the experience of continuity is the perception that providers know what has happened before, that different providers agree on a management plan, and that a provider who knows them will care for them in the future. For providers, the experience of continuity relates to their perception that they have sufficient knowledge and information about a patient to best apply their professional competence, and they have the confidence that their care inputs will be recognised and pursued by other providers.

*From Haggerty JL, Reid RJ, Freeman, GK, Starfield BH, Adair, CE, McKendry R. Continuity of care: a multidisciplinary review. *BMJ* 2003;327:1219-21

Useful material on websites

- To read about the information strategy of the UK NHS see www.nhsia.nhs.uk/def/pages/info4health/contents.asp
- Background reading and justification on proposed record keeping standards can be found at http://hiu.rcplondon.ac.uk/clinicalstandards/recordsstandards/index.asp
- The Ottawa Health Research Institute inventory of validated decision rules can be accessed at www.ohri.ca/programs/clinical_epidemiology/OHDEC/clinical.asp

---

Further reading

- Berwick DM. A primer on leading the improvement of systems. *BMJ* 1996;312:619-22
- Gardner M. Why clinical information standards matter. *BMJ* 2003;326:1101-2
- Wasson JH, Sox HC. Clinical prediction rules: have they come of age? *JAMA* 1996;275:641-2
- Wyatt JC, Altman DG. Prognostic models: clinically useful, or quickly forgotten? *BMJ* 1995;311:1539-41
- Schatz M, Cook EF, Joshua A, Petitti D. Risk factors for asthma hospitalizations in a managed care organization: development of a clinical prediction rule. *Am J Manag Care* 2003;9:538-47
- Guthrie B, Wyke S. Does continuity in general practice really matter? *BMJ* 2000;321:734-6
- Bates DW, Kuperman GJ, Wang S, Gandhi T, Kittler A, Volk L, et al. Ten commandments for effective clinical decision support: making the practice of evidence-based medicine a reality. *J Am Med Inform Assoc* 2003;10:523-30

8 Referral or follow-up?

When patients ask their doctors if a preventable problem could have been avoided by earlier investigation or referral, the doctors can be in an unenviable position. Given the information available at the time, the response will often be a qualified, "yes." It must be a qualified response because the aspects of the problem considered during earlier encounters with patients are often unknown. The matter is further complicated by issues of trust, professional ethics, and the law.

This article discusses information flows that may have reduced the risk of Ms Smith (see box opposite) developing symptomatic renal impairment. The risk could have been reduced at three different points.
- If her underlying vesicoureteric reflux had been diagnosed and fully investigated in childhood
- When her chronic pyelonephritis was discovered
- During the intervening period when no follow-up was arranged.

Early detection of underlying problems

Children aged ≤7 years with urinary symptoms, fever, or several non-specific symptoms and signs should be tested for urinary infections because, in some circumstances, prophylaxis can prevent recurrence. Guidelines are available, but the research that underpins the advice was published too late for Ms Smith. Were Ms Smith a young girl today, any primary care or emergency clinician who saw her would probably have access to this evidence base as part of their clinical software, or through access to guidelines on the internet.

Undergraduate education, postgraduate training, and continuing professional development are more traditional routes of knowledge transfer. Unfortunately, traditional sources of knowledge are relatively inefficient: our stores of knowledge decay over time, and our brain's working memory may become overloaded. Prompts and reminders at the point of care are useful adjuncts to an overworked human brain for certain tasks. Some doctors worry that use of such electronic aids may reduce patient trust, but the evidence is to the contrary.

Ensuring appropriate investigation

Fifteen years ago, when Ms Smith's chronic pyelonephritis was diagnosed, her investigation would probably have been directed by a consultant whose experience would have ensured the appropriate level of expertise was achieved. In the informatics age, some of this expertise can be represented in protocols. If the protocols are followed, investigation in primary care may avoid referral or identify the nature of the problem quickly and clearly. In some health systems, referring clinicians may be given shorter waiting lists if the referrals have been preceded by appropriate first line investigation.

Arranging referral

Health maintenance organisations in the United States, which provide integrated primary and secondary care, can book electronic appointments routinely. More complex referral settings may have difficulty doing this. Delays can occur at any

> Ms Smith is a 58 year old florist with a 15 year history of renal impairment caused by childhood pyelonephritis. She has hypercalcaemia. She remembers being told in the past that she had "a slight kidney problem," and asks her renal physician whether anything could have been done then to prevent the current problem developing

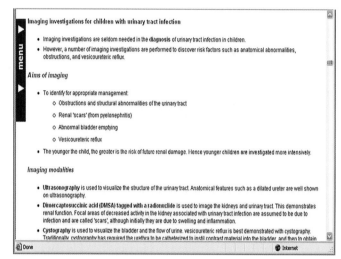

PRODIGY (Prescribing RatiOnally with Decision Support) guideline on investigation of urinary tract infection in children

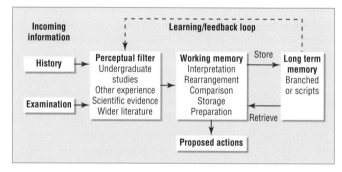

A model of human clinical information processing

Steps in the NHS process for non-urgent referral
- During a consultation the general practitioner (GP) considers if referral is appropriate
- Decision is negotiated, to a greater or lesser extent, with patient
- Decision and relevant clinical information is communicated to consultant or other secondary care provider, usually by letter
- Letter is posted or faxed to hospital
- Consultant prioritises referral
- Outpatient administrator allocates an appointment depending on the level of priority and the availability of appointments
- Appointment is communicated to patient, usually by letter
- Patient attends outpatient clinic and sees consultant or a member of their team

stage between the decision to refer and its realisation, even when an appointment is available.

Arranging follow-up

At the end of a hospital outpatient visit a decision is made about whether hospital, a GP, or shared care is most appropriate for the patient. Unless an arrangement is made the patient may have a "collusion of anonymity." This occurs when personnel at the hospital think that staff at the primary care practice are providing follow-up and vice versa. In reality, neither are doing so. To avoid such errors, healthcare systems have developed ways of integrating multiple service providers and proactive measures (see chronic care model opposite).

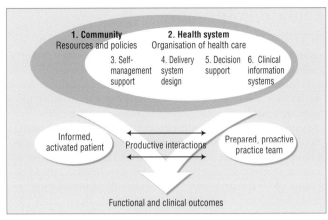

Overview of the chronic care model. Adapted from Wagner EH. *Effective Clin Pract* 1998;1:2-4

Hospital follow-up
When a consultant decides that a patient's problem needs hospital resources the flows of information are straightforward, but potential exists for errors and omissions. Often, patients are asked to book their next appointment as they leave the clinic. Alternatively, one of the clinic team may make the arrangement on the patient's behalf, and inform them at the time or by post.

> **If follow-up at hospital is needed then direct booking of the next visit avoids some potential difficulties**

GP follow-up
If the hospital team decide that the patient requires medical supervision, but no other hospital resources, the primary care team may be asked to resume sole responsibility for care. This is the simplest option for hospitals because it only needs a discharge letter to be sent. Most practices in the United Kingdom and other industrialised countries have the technology and systems to support a call-recall system for screening. Although this can be extended to support GP follow-up of chronic diseases, few practices are able to harness such systems to long term clinical care. This will probably change in countries like the United Kingdom, where achieving targets is increasingly important.

Shared care
Although shared care seems the most complex of the three follow-up options, done properly, it may be the best for the patient. An integrated service takes responsibility for all patients with the problem it is set up to deal with. Specialists ensure that healthcare services are configured to respond effectively to patients with problems, and to support clinicians working in the community.

Antenatal care is an example of this approach. Other areas of care, such as chronic diseases, are following suit, with excellent results seen in the care of people with diabetes and cardiovascular disease. Good, but often asynchronous, communication between colleagues with complementary skills is vital. In some systems, records may be seen by clinicians irrespective of where they are working.

Sharing information across health systems. Clinical data (for example, data on prescribing or blood pressure) in one part of the health system that have been recorded in primary care can be made available to other users, such as hospital clinicians, on a "need to know" basis

Patient empowerment

"Expert patients" have always been with us, but some doctors were not aware of it, or would not acknowledge it. No matter what arrangement is made for follow-up by the health professions, patients with chronic illnesses must deal with it every day. Better use of information helps, and consultations should be patient centred (to deal with patients' ideas, concerns, and expectations), but also extend beyond the visit.

> **Many doctors give patients an audiotape of their consultation, written material about their problem, or website addresses that provide further information. Others (hospital consultants, for example), may copy letters sent to GPs as text messages to the patient's mobile phone or send the letters to the patient as email attachments**

Clinical governance

As a result of apparent failures to ensure adequate patient care, society has demanded that arrangements for the supervision of clinical services are improved. The days of autonomy and paternalism are being replaced by rigorous inspection procedures and publication of results. Clinical teams need to show that they are working to the highest standards. This depends on their access to the best evidence about the criteria of good care and the standards that can be attained. Data, often from patient records, are then collected to confirm whether standards are being met, or if there are any defects to treasure. Failure to hit the target (for example, to offer annual blood pressure and renal function tests to Ms Smith), is an opportunity to improve the service. Electronic records make most of the service automatic, provided that patients agree to (or at least do not refuse) the secondary use of their personal data. Clinical teams can concentrate on providing a service, and using the information that has been captured (and processed) electronically to improve patient care. In the United Kingdom, the quality and outcomes framework of the new general medical services contract for GPs relies heavily on the electronic processing of Read coded data in clinical systems.

Summary

Achieving effective data transfer and electronic continuity of care between different parts of a health service is not essentially a technical challenge, rather it is a cultural and political one. It is largely about reconfiguring workflow. In 2004, the Veterans Health Administration showed that integrating clinical records across geographically and clinically diverse sites is feasible and valuable. Linking individual electronic patient records from different locations into a single electronic health record will probably transform the quality of health services over the next decade.

UK general practice contract quality points for management of hypertension

Indicator	Coverage	Points
Register of patients	Yes/no	9
Smoking status	25-90%	10
Smoking advice	25-90%	10
Blood pressure recorded in past 9 months	25-90%	20
Blood pressure ≤ 150/90 mm Hg	25-70%	56

Further reading

- Williams GJ, Lee A, Craig JC. Long-term antibiotics for preventing recurrent urinary tract infection in children. *Cochrane Database Syst Rev* 2001;4:CD001534

- The diagnosis, treatment, and evaluation of the initial urinary tract infection in febrile infants and young children: www.guideline.gov/summary/summary.aspx?doc_id = 1838&nbr = 1064&ss = 6 (accessed 19 October 2005)

- Sullivan FM, MacNaughton RJ. Evidence used in consultations: interpreted and individualised. *Lancet* 1996;348:941-3

- Hunt DL, Haynes B, Hanna SE, Smith K. Effects of computer-based clinical decision support systems on physician performance and patient outcomes. A systematic review. *JAMA* 1998;280:1339-46

- Wagner EH. Chronic disease management: What will it take to improve care for chronic illness? *Effective Clin Pract* 1998;1:2-4

- NHS Confederation. General Medical Services contract negotiations: www.nhsconfed.org/gmscontract/ (accessed 19 October 2005)

- Perlin JB, Kolodner RM, Roswell RH. The Veterans Health Administration: quality, value, accountability, and information as transforming strategies for patient-centered care. *Am J Manag Care* 2004;10:828-36

9 Keeping up: learning in the workplace

The amount of biomedical knowledge doubles every 20 years, and new classes of drug (such as phosphodiesterase 4 inhibitors) become available when lectures at medical school are over. Therefore, a practice risks fossilising after doctors finish professional training. Many continuing medical education or continuing professional development activities help doctors carry on learning and improving their skills. These activities include courses, conferences, mailed educational materials, weekly grand rounds, journal clubs, and using internet sites. In many countries, evidence of this process is needed for doctors to continue to practice. Although these activities may increase knowledge, their impact on clinical practice is variable

The aim of traditional medical education is to commit knowledge to memory and then use this knowledge in the workplace. The way knowledge is learnt influences its recall and application to work. One tactic to improve the process is to ensure that learning happens in the clinical workplace. Lessons are learnt faster and recalled more reliably when they originate in everyday experience.

Learning in the workplace means spending a minute here or three minutes there to find answers prompted by the clinical questions and learning opportunities that come up in every working day, rather than doing continuing medical education for an intensive two hours a week, or a few days a year. Workplace learning is hard to achieve. It emphasises problem solving and learning skills—such as how to find relevant answers fast—not learning facts.

Barriers and solutions

Nobody can find a satisfactory answer to every clinical question or information need, especially as there are about two needs for every three clinical encounters. Many important clinical questions have no satisfactory answer—for example, what is the cause of motor neurone disease? Other questions are simply interesting rather than information needs. A range of practical difficulties face doctors who follow the approach of learning in the workplace. Some suggestions about how to overcome the difficulties follow.

Too many questions, not enough time

Doctors generate approximately 45 questions about patient care every week, and they probably allow two minutes to answer each one. This adds up to an extra hour and a half per week, and even though it represents only 3% of their working time, where do doctors find this time? Time is always short. They often have to adjust the threshold for seeking answers, prioritising questions that have the highest clinical impact and are quickest to answer.

Prioritising clinical questions by the likely impact of the answer means distinguishing between the questions in the box opposite. When doctors have time, they can pursue all answers. When under pressure, they pursue answers that are needed now (category 1). If they never pursue other answers, they will miss many clinical advances. It is often hard to recognise when knowledge is lacking, and so it is important to sometimes pursue answers even when only slightly uncertain of the answer.

> **Patrick Murphy is a 6 year old boy who has recently returned home from a hospital admission. The discharge letter asks you to prescribe inhaled steroids and a phosphodiesterase 4 inhibitor**

> **Workplace learning means finding solutions to clinical problems when they arise, or soon after, with minimum effort. When unsure about what has happened, why, or what to do, answers should be looked up**

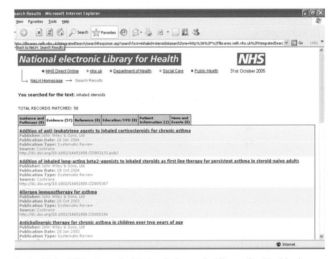

In the United Kingdom, the National electronic Library for Health aims to provide answers within 15 seconds that take only 15 seconds to read

Prioritisation of clinical questions

1 Answers needed now
2 Answers needed before patient is seen next
3 Answers needed to guide care of other patients or to reorganise clinical practice
4 Answers that have interest to doctor and patient, but carry no obvious clinical impact

To ease time pressure, clinicians can spend less time answering a question by using knowledge resources that are comprehensive, and can be instantly accessed and easily searched. They could also increase the time available for workplace learning. Individually, doctors can work for longer hours, reserving time for "reflective practice" with a preceptor or mentor, exploiting "teachable moments," perhaps by answering an educational prescription. Overall, the medical profession needs to recognise the sanctity of workplace learning throughout doctors' careers: life long, self directed learning.

Lack of clear questions

Asking clear questions is not easy. Sometimes doctors feel uncertain and fail to formalise a question, which makes it harder to find the answer. Immediate identification of clinical questions is important, and is easiest to do on ward rounds or when teaching students. When working alone, some clinicians log their questions (for example, on BMJLearning), then look up the learning resources on the website (the "just in time learning" package on childhood asthma) or other sources, or they discuss the answer with peers later. Structuring clinical questions using the problem, intervention, comparison and outcome (PICO) model makes them easier to focus, recall, and answer.

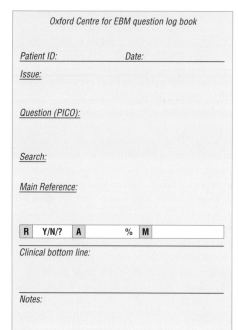

Adapted from a page from the Oxford Centre for Evidence Based Medicine's logbook (R=randomised and representative, A=ascertainment or follow-up rate percentage, M=measures unbiased, relevant)

Turning clinical problems into easily investigated formats

	Patient or problem	Intervention (or cause, prognostic factor, treatment)	Comparison (if necessary)	Outcomes
Tips for building	Starting with your patient ask "How would I describe a group of patients similar to mine?" Balance precision with brevity	Ask "Which main intervention am I considering?" Be specific	Ask "What is the main alternative to compare with the intervention?" Be specific	Ask "What can I hope to accomplish?" or "What could this exposure really affect?" Be specific
Example (see scenario on p 25)	In children with poorly controlled asthma …	"… would adding phosphodiesterase 4 inhibitor to inhaled corticosteroid …"	"… when compared with adding a long acting ß agonist …"	"… reduce the likelihood of readmission?"

Lack of answers

A source of answers needs to be available in the workplace. This source should provide answers that are clinically relevant, scientifically sound, and in a form that can influence decisions. One solution is a library in the workplace that contains current text and reference books, relevant reprints, and electronic resources. The library must be close and organised for rapid access. The material should be filtered for clinical relevance and be evidence based, such as *Clinical Evidence* in book or CD-Rom format or an indexed collection of systematic reviews.

These sources will not answer all questions. In Patrick Murphy's case (see scenario on p 25) the treatment is not indexed, and so online access to Medline will be needed, preferably via the PubMed clinical queries search page that provides answers useful to practicing doctors. Ideally, doctors will then retrieve the full text of relevant articles because relying on the abstract alone can be misleading. When Pitkin compared the statements made in 264 structured abstracts in six medical journals with the corresponding article, a fifth contained statements that were not substantiated in the article and 28% contained statements that disagreed with those in the article. Thus, tempting though it may be to rely on abstracts alone—especially because they are now so accessible through PubMed—it can be dangerous.

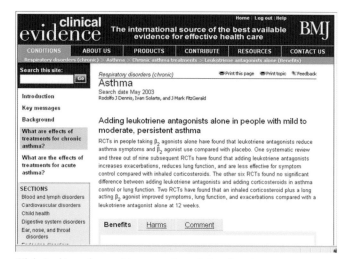

Clinical evidence is a useful resource in workplace learning

An alternative to carrying out the search yourself is to call or email a question answering service, such as ATTRACT, for clinicians working in Wales. For years, NHS poisons and drug information services have provided similar services that give instant answers to specialist questions. Some libraries, primary care trusts and academic departments have services that cover many topics. The service usually returns a telephone call or sends a summary within two to four hours. Despite their obvious potential, these services seem underused at present.

Parochialism

If doctors only look up answers to questions arising in their own practice, their knowledge will depend on the local case mix. Most doctors broaden their knowledge by reading a general medical journal or looking up points raised in replies to referrals, inpatient summaries, clinic letters, or laboratory reports. Some participate in multidisciplinary clinics or ward rounds, or join colleagues in an email discussion group. To be ready for rare, serious problems that need an instant response, some clinicians use patient simulators to practice managing cardiopulmonary arrest, anaesthetic accidents, or brittle diabetes. Although time spent on simulators does not yet count towards doctors' continuing education, taking part in interactive cases in some journals does.

Lack of incentives

To maintain the enthusiasm to keep looking up answers to clinical questions, doctors can keep a log book of questions and answers, or conduct clinical audits that compare practice and outcomes with results a year ago. Such log books and audit reports will become part of doctors' folders for accreditation and annual appraisal.

Sharing insights is an incentive to learn, and giving a presentation often prompts discussion, especially if it is short, and it defines and deals with a real clinical problem (along with sources searched, the answers found, and actions taken). This activity can be formalised as a single page, dated, critically appraised topic (CAT), and stored in a loose leaf folder or a practice intranet for others.

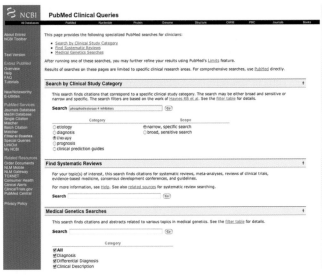

A PubMed search filters for clinical queries

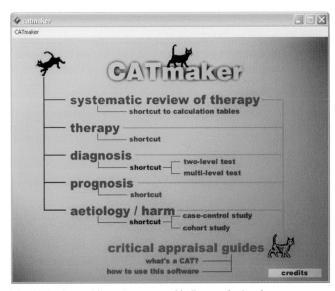

The CATmaker tool is used to create critically appraised topics

---

Cultural changes associated with workplace learning

Old think	New think
• Passive listening to lectures	• Active participation in self directed learning
• Educator decides topic	• You decide topic
• Attend continuing medical education course you know most about	• Seek out areas of ignorance and answers to your clinical questions
• Focus is on laboratory research, pathophysiology, drug mechanisms	• Focus is on what works in practice, what to do, problem solving
• Read a journal or textbook	• Carry out problem solving on real or simulated cases
• Education to learn facts, pass exams	• Learning to solve clinical problems, improve team work, clinical and information seeking skills
• Formal, timed courses	• Informal, self directed, learning in the workplace
• Get continuing medical education or postgraduate education allowance points for turning up	• Get continuing medical education or postgraduate education allowance points for participating in workplace learning, using learning materials, improving standards
• Case presentation, journal club	• Work on an educational prescription, write a critically appraised topic, use a clinical simulator
• Competition: keep knowledge to yourself	• Sharing: open learning, exchange of knowledge and understanding to benefit patients and the health system
• Knowledge belongs to the individual. Continuing medical education points accumulate to the individual. Recertify the individual	• Communities of practice: learning is an attribute of the team and organisation and is part of its quality and risk management strategies. Accredit the organisation
• Patients are passive recipients of care	• Patients are sources of questions and insights, learning collaborators
• Errors should be forgotten and denied	• Errors are a learning experience to be treasured, discussed, and understood
• Errors happen to "bad apples"	• Errors happen to everyone

Lowering barriers is also motivating: an old *BNF* in a desk drawer will be used more often than a current version in the practice library 10 m away, or one in the health library 5 km away. Electronic libraries and the internet bring the world's literature to your desktop, but can take longer and yield fewer answers to clinical questions than paper sources. This is changing. A German study found that clinical use of online learning was about ten times that of print journals.

Summary

Barriers to workplace learning can be overcome, but a minor culture change in the medical profession is needed. This shift is already taking place in undergraduate medical education and in primary care. Clinical governance, risk management, patient empowerment, and the National Programme for IT will further advance the change.

Using clinical questions to guide workplace learning relies on the motivation of individuals, teams, and organisations. It goes hand in hand with an open attitude to clinical errors and near misses. Motivation is especially necessary to fund the instant access resources needed to provide knowledge during clinical work. Fortunately, electronic media provide a simpler, cheaper method for workplace learning than paper libraries, although there is evidence that health librarians on site are still needed to support better clinical use of these resources.

Further reading

- Wyatt J. Use and sources of medical knowledge. *Lancet* 1991;338:1368-73
- General Medical Council. *A licence to practice and revalidation.* London: General Medical Council, 2003
- Mazmanian PE, Davis DA. Continuing medical education and the physician as a learner: guide to the evidence. *JAMA* 2002;288:1057-60
- Lave J, Wenger E. *Situated learning.* Cambridge: Cambridge University Press, 1991
- Ebell MH, Shaughnessy A. Information mastery: integrating continuing medical education with the information needs of clinicians. *J Contin Educ Health Prof* 2003;23:53-62
- The resourceful patient website. The e-consultation: vignette. www.resourcefulpatient.org/resources/econsult.htm (accessed 30 October 2005)
- Smith R. What clinical information do doctors need? *BMJ* 1996; 313:1062-8
- Ely JW, Osheroff JA, Ebell MH, Chambliss ML, Vinson DC, Stevermer JJ, et al. Obstacles to answering doctors' questions about patient care with evidence: qualitative study. *BMJ* 2002;324:710
- PubMed clinical queries: www.ncbi.nlm.nih.gov/entrez/query/ static/clinical.html (accessed 30 October 2005)
- Pitkin RM, Branagan MA, Burmeister LF. Accuracy of data in abstracts of published research articles. *JAMA* 1999; 281:1110-11
- ATTRACT: www.attract.wales.nhs.uk/index.cfm (accessed 30 October 2005)
- Harker N, Montgomery A, Fahey T. Treating nausea and vomiting during pregnancy: case outcome. *BMJ* 2004;328:503

10 Improving services with informatics tools

This article describes how many sources of data can be linked, interpreted, and analysed before being presented to decision makers to improve care. It also discusses the legal issues surrounding data protection and freedom of information.

A huge volume of data flows across the desk of a director of public health (see box opposite). One of the director's problems is to know which signals to act upon and what "noise" to ignore. If the numbers being considered are small, as they probably will be in the case described here, a critical incident analysis may be all that is needed. An individual prescriber, or group, may have an erroneous belief or inadequate training. Critical incidents or other signals often indicate that more data (such as data on prescribing steroids for paediatric asthma in primary care and outpatients) are needed.

Sources of data

Health services are awash with data. Earlier articles in the series described the large and increasing numbers of sources of data available to consumers, patients, clinicians, and administrators. Clinicians, teams, divisions, and other groups collect the data they need to carry out their work, and they may do so using coding and terms that others can understand and share. The intensive care unit in this example integrated the data the team needs to manage patients during their stay with patients' pre-admission prescribing data. This local epidemiology may have been done as part of clinical governance activities, or as an ad hoc exercise when a patient's problem was investigated.

One difficulty with secondary uses of clinical data is that, having obtained the data indicating a problem exists, the issue must be dealt with effectively. It may be that the individual or group who identify the problem have the knowledge, skills, and resources to resolve it. In other cases, such as these potentially avoidable asthma admissions, those responsible are not those who have uncovered the issue, and those potentially responsible may be unaware of the problem.

Presentation of data

Ideally, the choice of measures, analysis, and presentation of data should be determined by the purpose of measurement and the use to which data are to be put. This poses another difficulty with the secondary use of clinical data. Studies have shown that interpretation of data is influenced by the method used to summarise the results. Health policy makers, like doctors, tend to prefer measurements that report relative risks (or benefits) to measurements providing estimates of absolute risks (or benefits). Once the decision has been taken to act on data, how best to present the information should be considered.

Feedback of performance data

Different approaches (using internal or external influences on decision makers) can be taken when using data to improve care. The interventions chosen should be tailored to the underlying problem. At least two, and preferably three, of the more effective approaches (see boxes on next page) should be taken.

You are a director of public health. The local paediatric intensive care unit sends you a paper describing five potentially avoidable admissions in the past two years—for example, patients with severe asthma who were not being prescribed prophylactic drugs

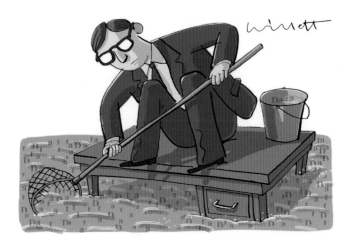

UK clinical governance definition*

A framework through which NHS organisations are accountable for continually improving the quality of their services and safeguarding high standards of care by creating an environment in which excellence in clinical care will flourish

*From Scally G, Donaldson LJ. Clinical governance and the drive for quality improvement in the new NHS in England. *BMJ* 1998;317:61-5

Categories of improvement for health services*

- Safety
- Effectiveness
- Patient centredness
- Timeliness
- Efficiency
- Equity

*From Institute of Medicine Committee on Quality of Health Care in America.*Crossing the quality chasm: a new health system for the 21st century.* Washington, DC: National Academy Press, 2001

Analysis of approaches to changing clinical practice: internal processes*

Approach	Theories	Focus	Interventions, strategy
Educational	Adult learning theories	Intrinsic motivation of professionals	Bottom up, local consensus development Small group interactive learning Problem based learning
Epidemiological	Cognitive theories	Rational information seeking and decision making	Evidence based guideline development Disseminating research findings through courses, mailing, journals
Marketing	Health promotion, innovation and social marketing theories	Attractive product adapted to needs of target audience	Needs assessment, adapting change proposals to local needs Stepwise approach Various channels for dissemination (mass media and personal)

Analysis of approaches to changing clinical practice: external processes*

Approach	Theories	Focus	Interventions, strategy
Behavioural	Learning theory	Controlling performance by external stimuli	Audit and feedback Reminder systems, monitoring Economic incentives, sanctions
Social interaction	Social learning and innovation theories, social influence and power theories	Social influence of important peers or role models	Peer review in local networks Outreach visits, individual instruction Opinion leaders Influencing key people in social networks Patient mediated interventions
Organisational	Management theories, system theories	Creating structural and organisational conditions to improve care	Re-engineering care process Total quality management and continuous quality improvement approaches Team building Enhancing leadership Changing structures, tasks
Coercive	Economic, power, and learning theories	Control and pressure, external motivation	Regulations, laws Budgeting, contracting Licensing, accreditation Complaints and legal procedures

*Reproduced from Grol R. Beliefs and evidence in changing clinical practice. *BMJ* 1997;315:418-21

Today, it is less necessary to rely on individual clinicians or teams to produce routine reports because computerised data entry enables the routine extraction of data for many purposes. Data from multiple sources may be linked to records, and so provide additional intelligence beyond the purposes for which they were originally collected.

Record linkage

Deterministic or probabilistic methods can be used with similar success rates to link records. In the former case, a unique patient identifier, such as a 10 digit community health index number, is applied to all personal health data—for example, laboratory test requests and prescriptions. In the latter case, algorithms determine the likelihood that two items of data belong to the same person. The Soundex system converts a name to a code (for example, Michael becomes M240). The first letter is the first letter of the word, and the numbers represent phonetic parts of latter syllables. The algorithm determines that John Smyth and John Smythe is the same child with asthma if sufficient other characteristics (date of birth, street name) on the admission data and community prescriptions match. After linkage, each individual item of data may then be linked and anonymised for disease surveillance purposes.

Data protection

The main provisions of the 1998 Data Protection Act were implemented on 1 March 2000. This act builds on the earlier 1984 Data Protection Act. It is the means whereby the United Kingdom enforces the 1995 European directive on data

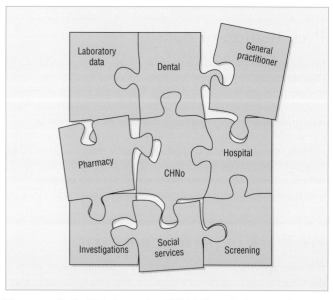

The community health index number (CHNo) is a unique 10 digit number that includes the date of birth of individuals born, or moving to, Scotland so that their encounters with the health service can be linked

The community health index number (CHNo) allows the fragmented episodes of care experienced by individuals to be integrated into the completed jigsaw of an electronic health record

protection. It aims to ensure that the processing (obtaining, recording, holding, doing calculations on) of information using data is done in accordance with the rights of individuals. The European directive also extends the legislation to manual, as well as computerised, records containing personal information. Under the provisions of the act, data controllers (for example, general practitioners) are responsible for ensuring that access to patient data should be under strictly controlled conditions and, if necessary, with patients' consent.

Eight principles of good practice are in the act. Patients should be aware, at least in broad terms, of the purposes for which their personal data are used. However, it is the view of the data protection registrar that consent should normally be obtained when processing data about a patient's health. Many Caldicott guardians believe that the activities of the NHS are often in the public interest, and in most cases the consent of the patient can be inferred. Other bodies, such as the General Medical Council and the BMA, advise that explicit consent is still preferable in some cases, and examples include:

- Release of details of patients to diabetic and cancer registers
- Release of summaries of patient date to out of hours services.

The 2000 Freedom of Information Act came into force in January 2005. It is intended to "promote a culture of openness and accountability amongst public sector bodies by providing people with rights of access to the information held by them." It will probably conflict with data protection legislation because information about individuals is contextualised within families, communities, practices, and hospital units. It will be difficult to ensure that an individual's data are protected while giving freedom of information to others within that context.

Feedback of information

In many medical cultures it is difficult to provide feedback that will be taken in a constructive manner. Certain principles make it more likely that the feedback will be considered constructive by recipients, and changes that could improve care will probably be implemented.

Research governance

Confidentiality and security of data is probably a greater concern for researchers than clinicians, although clinical researchers need to live with concept of governance in both worlds. Data collected for patient care may only be used to produce research evidence with adequate safeguards for the patients. Legislation varies between countries, but the highest standards apply to use of personally identifiable data, where explicit signed, informed consent is often required. Some jurisdictions relax this standard if it is impossible, or extremely difficult, to obtain the consent. In other countries acceptable anonymisation and adherence to rules of good epidemiological practice allow the use of clinical data for research purposes.

Summary

A public health consultant faced with complex, difficult choices, such as the data on asthma prescribing, will prefer to discuss the reasons for apparent prescribing failures rather than taking pre-emptive action, which may do harm to the service overall. The factors that caused the presenting problem are often rooted in the culture of the health system, and so the solution often means changing the system. The consequences of failing to act when there is a problem need to be counterbalanced against the damage caused by incorrect interpretation of data collected for one purpose but used for another.

Principles of good practice in the 1998 Data Protection Act

Data are:
- Fairly and lawfully processed
- Processed for limited purposes
- Adequate, relevant, and not excessive
- Accurate
- Not kept longer than necessary
- Processed in accordance with the rights of the subject of the data
- Secure
- Not transferred to countries without adequate protection

Dame FIONA Caldicott's principles of data processing*

- **F**ormal justification of purpose
- **I**nformation transferred only when absolutely necessary
- **O**nly the minimum required
- **N**eed to know access controls
- **A**ll to understand their responsibilities
- **C**omply with and understand the law

* http://pmj.bmjjournals.com/cgi/content/full/79/935/516

Approaches identified by the Nuffield Trust to deal with the conflict between the the Freedom of Information Act and data protection legislation

- Use personal data with consent or other assent from the subjects of the data
- Anonymise the data, then use them
- Use personal data without explicit consent, under a public interest mandate

---

Key issues in data feedback to improve quality*

- Data must be perceived by clinicians as valid to motivate change
- It takes time to develop the credibility of data
- The source and timeliness of data are critical to perceived validity
- Benchmarking improves the meaningfulness of data feedback
- Opinion leaders can enhance the effectiveness of data feedback
- Data feedback that profiles an individual clinician's practices can be effective but may be perceived as punitive
- Data feedback must persist to sustain improved performance

*Bradley EH, Holmboe ES, Mattera JA, Roumanis SA, Radford MJ, Krumholz HM. Data feedback efforts in quality improvement: lessons learned from US hospitals. *Qual Safety Health Care* 2004;13:26-31

Further reading

- Grimshaw JM, Thomas RE, MacLennan G, Fraser C, Ramsay CR, Vale L, et al. Effectiveness and efficiency of guideline dissemination and implementation strategies. *Health Technol Assess* 2004;8:1-72
- NHS Health Technology Assessment Programme. Effectiveness and efficiency of guideline dissemination and implementation strategies: www.ncchta.org/execsumm/summ806.htm (accessed 4 October)
- Fahey T, Griffiths S, Peters TJ. Evidence based purchasing: understanding results of clinical trials and systematic reviews. *BMJ* 1995;311:1056-9
- Lowrence WW. *"Learning from experience." Privacy and the secondary uses of data.* London: The Nuffield Trust, 2002
- Berwick DM. Errors today and errors tomorrow. *N Engl J Med* 2003;348:2570-72

11 Communication and navigation around the healthcare system

However good a doctor's clinical skills, record keeping abilities, and mastery of evidence, before they can start work they need directory information. This is the information patients and professionals use to find their way around the healthcare system. Different grades of staff have different demands for this information, and all staff are often interrupted by colleagues' requests for this information.

> You are a general practice locum and need to fix an outpatient assessment for Mrs Smith's bronchitis. The receptionist mentions that before you organise the assessment you need to book certain tests that vary according to which chest physician you refer Mrs Smith to. The receptionist does not know the names of local chest physicians nor their investigation preferences. You spend 15 minutes trying to call the chest clinic in the nearest hospital before discovering it moved six weeks ago to another site 15 miles (24 km) away. Your phone is not cleared for long distance calls, and the practice manager is not around, so you wait to use a colleague's phone. Mrs Smith takes umbrage at the delay and walks out while shouting across the waiting room, "Call yourself a doctor. You don't even know what goes on in the hospitals round here."

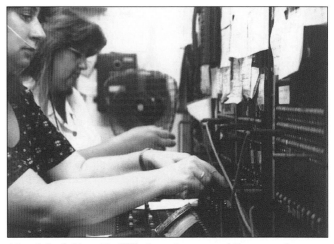

A hospital switchboard in 1995—shows the operators' directory and temporary notes. With permission from Martin Loach

Directory information

Directory information includes information about local services, how to book them, contact details, and specialists' preferences for tests that they need patients to have had done before they see them. Variations in stationery, laboratory and therapeutic services, and how those services are organised (including what type of bottle specimens should go in) mean that most expert clinicians cannot work properly when they are moved from their base 100 km in any direction.

Initiatives from the national programme for information technology (NPfIT), such as "Choose and book" with its electronic directories of specialists and their preferences for which tests should be done before a patient is referred, should provide a few types of directory information.

Communication

Directory information has always been needed. In the past, doctors could rely on informal networks built up over years, and there were fewer subspecialists to swell clinical teams. Now, health systems change more often, members of staff are more mobile, and the scope of health has widened so that doctors regularly communicate with local authorities, expert patients, carers, a variety of hospitals, and voluntary agencies. Also, the number of staff in each health centre has increased.

Although new technologies may reduce the need for doctors to memorise information, they raise new problems—for example, access to a directory is needed to check qualifications of remote telecarers and identify them reliably so that doctors can hand over responsibilities and information to them.

Little is known about the patterns of communication within and beyond clinical teams, although interesting results have

Directory information used to support primary care tasks

Primary care task	Directory information	Source
Routine surgical referral	List of surgeons with interests and waiting times at local hospitals	Colleagues, human resources department at local acute trust, trust website, Dr Foster
Urgent psychiatric referral	Telephone number of local mental health trust, person on duty and their mobile number	*Hospital and Health Services Yearbook*, local mental health trust
Therapy referral	List of therapists by location, days they work, and their contact details	Local primary care trust
Test ordering	Type of specimen, tube needed, suggested indications	Local laboratory handbook
Test interpretation	Reference range, who to call for advice	Local laboratory handbook
Advice to patients	For example, details of local diabetes self help group, or details of an Asperger's self help group	Primary care trust, Diabetes UK website, Contact-a-Family website
Inquiry about new general practice contract	List of local primary care priorities	Primary care trust headquarters
Writing job description for practice manager	Salary scales	BMA regional adviser

emerged from a small study of hospital communication and a study of emails sent between primary care centres and trusts. The best evidence for taking a proactive approach to managing communication comes from the field of mental health.

Studies of case workers show the benefit of a formal approach to exchanging information when dealing with a complex chronic disease that has a relapsing and remitting time course. To understand what happens during communication between different parts of a health system, reflect on the main elements of any communication. It requires at least two parties (sender and receiver) who share some similar understanding of the world (common ground). Communication also needs a message, which may be short and simple, or complex (such as a drug formulary), and a channel over which the message can travel. Communication channels can vary in important ways. Some channels require the simultaneous attention of both parties (for example, face to face conversations), other channels automatically provide a permanent record of the message (for example, faxes or emails). In any communication, the person whom the message is for, and the nature of the message must be established. In some situations, such as the scenario in the box on page 32, assembling and using reliable directory information is difficult.

Collecting and using directory information

Collecting and using such information can be difficult for several reasons. Clinicians rely heavily on printed lists and handbooks. This hard copy often needs to be corrected or annotated, and then photocopied because some staff cannot access the original electronic copy. Another reason for there being problems with collecting and using directory information is that clinicians often rely on their fallible memories. Fragmentation of information sources can also cause difficulties. Sometimes work related contact numbers are stored in diaries or mobile phones, and either could be lost or stolen. Also, if stored in a phone or diary, this information is not automatically available to others in the healthcare team or beyond.

NHS HealthSpace (www.healthspace.nhs.uk) allows patients to record these data. Patients can store their own information in the section called "Health Tracker," and will have access to their electronic health records.

External agencies often manage directory information better than the NHS. For example, Binley's directory provides information from contact details for NHS trusts, departments, and health centres, to pharmacy opening times. Private healthcare organisations also manage information better than the NHS because they realise that there is a business need and that benefits will accrue if their clients have easy access to information on how to use their services.

Assembling, maintaining, and accessing directory information

One of the reasons that any clinician could face a situation like the one described in the scenario is because the people and organisations in healthcare services change fast. In the future they will change even faster, making directory information more important, but more difficult to assemble.

Communication channels used in healthcare

Channel	Sender and receiver needed at same time	Type and longevity of record	Comment
Face to face conversation	Yes	Usually none, but can be partial or full	Can make notes later, tape record whole encounter
Telephone conversation	Yes	Usually none, but can be partial or full	Can make notes during or after, or record in full for permanent record (for example, NHSDirect)
Voicemail	No	None or temporary	Can delete or save for 28 days
Text messages	No	None or temporary, or can be full	Can archive text messages permanently
Email	No	Permanent	Can forward to others and attach pictures
Instant messaging	Nearly, reply needed within a minute	Permanent	Can save chat to disk
Ward round	Yes	Partial	Record findings and decisions in case notes
Meeting	Yes (even if done by telephone or video)	Partial	Minutes of meeting
Telemedicine using store and forward	No	Permanent	Similar to email
Telemedicine using video link	Yes	Usually none, but can be partial or full	Like a ward round. Record results and decisions in case notes, or video record the session
Interactive digital television	Yes	No	Slow with poor functionality, but will improve
Exchange of letters or fax	No	Yes	Older technologies that have a continuing role

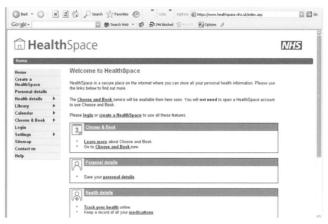

NHS HealthSpace website allows patients to store information and will allow them to private access to their personal electronic health records

Summary

Directory information is vital for people to navigate healthcare services and to allow clinicians to do their work, but in many healthcare organisations directory information is under-rated, or even non-existent.

Directory information changes quickly, and originates locally. It also needs to be accurate, up to date, and available nationally to support greater use of eHealth. Some of the information can be distilled from local sources of data, and one approach might be to expect it to be everyone's business to ensure that these sources are kept up to date—just as clinicians maintain a patient's record.

Unfortunately, this idea leads to a "collusion of anonymity" where "everyone agreed that someone should do it, but no one did." A solution might be to have a designated person for each organisation—for example, a laboratory or primary care centre—whose job it is to maintain this information. Maintaining directory information can be seen as "organisational governance." It is an intrinsic part of being a team member and central to being a responsible employee.

It seems ironic that when accurate, comprehensive, up to date contact information is needed by NHS organisations, they pay for directories and databases published by external organisations—for example, Binleys directory, NHS Confederation, and Medical Directory. Perhaps the NHS should outsource this activity and set up central service level agreements with these organisations for less money than NHS Trusts currently spend on paper directories. Pressure from an external contracted organisation might persuade organisations that are funded by the state to provide the necessary data in a timely way, which has often defeated internal efforts to capture these data in the past. In future, pre-referral investigation protocols for each consultant might be readily available and potential Mrs Smiths need not be so disappointed.

Further reading

- Coiera EW, Jayasuriya RA, Hardy J, Bannan A, Thorpe ME. Communication loads on clinical staff in the emergency department. *Med J Aust* 2002;176:415-8
- Coiera E, Tombs V. Communication behaviours in a hospital setting: an observational study. *BMJ* 1998;316:673-6
- Ziguras SJ, Stuart GW, Jackson AC. Assessing the evidence on case management. *Br J Psychiatry* 2002;181:17-21
- Coulter A. When I'm 64: Health choices. *Health Expect* 2004;7:95-7

Collecting and using directory information

Problem	Solution
Source of directory information is often obscure	Identify key data and most accurate source
It is nobody's job to maintain the source	Include directory information in information governance role
Too many sources, no coherent map	Map and reduce the number of sources
No single format for directory information	Develop a national standard data format for all relevant kinds of directory information
Cannot rely on peers or traditional networks in view of shorter working week, rapid staff changes	Use electronic media
Directory information changes fast—for example, contacts, laboratory tests, opening hours of pharmacy	Someone must keep it up to date on a central site; discourage print outs
Maintaining accurate, up to date contact information takes a lot of work	Reward those who succeed by including it in their job description
Most directories are designed for local users in a local context, but data increasingly needed at national level	Ensure national standard format, context seen as national not local
Local NHS regularly reorganised	Include directory information management as a function in every new organisation; anticipate and manage risks of disruption
Plurality of NHS service provision—private sector, overseas, other providers	Encourage all service providers to use and contribute to NHS directory information
Disruption to work caused by use of synchronous communication channels	Encourage use of asynchronous channels instead by providing email or voicemail details
Loss of key directory information caused by use of transient channels, such as mobile phones, Post It notes	Use permanent channels
Print outs of electronic copy get out of date, and corrections are rarely propagated	Do not print out
Data in diary or handheld computer is hidden from other team members and can get lost	Download data, never modify it on handheld computer
Variable quality of NHS directory information	Raise awareness of importance of directory information; use it; allow users to improve it; outsource capture and provision of other providers

12   eHealth and the future: promise or peril?

Despite the futuristic sound of the scenario in the box below, all the technologies mentioned are available, and some, such as computer interviewing, have been used since the 1960s.

Such a scenario raises questions about the nature of clinical practice and healthcare systems—for example, how much information and responsibility should be transferred to patients when technology allows it. This final article examines some of these issues, and ends the series where it started, with a reminder that health informatics is more about understanding people and new models of care than it is about technology.

Factors encouraging eHealth

Gustafson and Wyatt define eHealth as "patients and the public using the internet or other electronic media to disseminate or provide access to health and lifestyle information or services." This differs from telemedicine, in which there is a health professional at one or both ends of the communication.

Pressures towards the use of eHealth include:
- Patient demand—Information and services can be delivered in a personalised way, where and when they are wanted. eHealth provides simple, easy access to health information, support services, and goods. It can lead to loss of the general practitioner's role as mediator (for example, a patient and specialist could email each other directly) and enhanced self expression (for example, in weblogs)
- New functions—eHealth can link previously distinct services and information. For example, all the information and forms from different government departments relevant to having a baby could be accessed from one portal
- Democracy—eHealth could allow citizens to form pressure groups, lobby for services, or even set up their own health organisations (see box at bottom of page 36)
- Health workforce—eHealth may help deal with staff shortages or requests from staff for improved working lives (for example, working from home)
- Technology—Futuristic devices (like implanted sensors and drug delivery systems) are made possible as technology becomes more reliable, functional, and cheaper
- National policy—eHealth could help move towards services that are better coordinated, promote equity and patient independence, and adhere to government targets and lower carbon dioxide emissions (eHealth favours home based care)
- Economics—eHealth shifts some costs to the patient or community
- Safety—For example, eHealth may allow improved self management and avoidance of exposure to methicillin resistant *Staphylococcus aureus* (MRSA).

It is 2014 and Mrs Smith has ongoing trouble with her high blood pressure. One morning she wakes with a headache and worries that the reservoir of her implanted drug delivery system may be running down. Her bedside ambient health orb (see www.ambientdevices.com) is a reassuring green, but she turns to her video wall and asks "Cyberdoc, how are my recent blood pressure levels?" The simulated voice responds "Your records show that the drug reservoir needs a refill in three weeks time. Your telemetered blood pressure readings have been under control for the past month and today's figures are normal. Your implanted blood sugar sensor shows normal readings too. Do you have some symptoms that you want to discuss?" Meanwhile Mrs Smith's wall graphs her recent blood pressure readings, and a list of the most common 20 symptoms affecting people of her age group in the locality. She responds, "No, don't worry. Remind me to book my repeat prescription (for a refill) in two weeks, please."

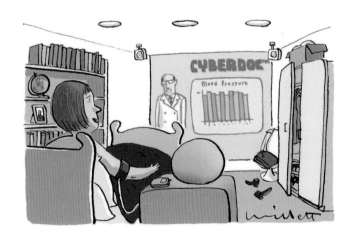

How will eHealth develop?

In the short term, general practice and hospital websites may evolve from passive "brochure ware" (practice information and general patient advice) to active ecommerce-like applications that allow information exchange and transactions. So, general practice websites may soon cater for patients, carers, and others by providing the facilities listed on page 36.

Potential benefits of developments in eHealth

- Better information and choice for patients, carers, and others
- Better communication of patient information to and between primary care team, leading to fewer phone calls, appointments, and improved adherence to treatment

- Links to external sites that have been selected for quality—for example, patient support organisations and leaflets
- A secure personal page for each patient providing access to their official medical record, including their lists of drugs, results of tests, copies of letters, and discharge summaries
- A link to NHS HealthSpace, which allows patients to construct their own "health biography," and enter data about long term conditions, rather than using a diary card
- Forms to book appointments or request repeat prescriptions
- A secure structured clinical enquiry form to capture patient symptoms and prompt a response from a general practitioner (GP) in the requested time.

Personal agents

Personal agents (also known as multiagent systems) are a technology that may enable patients to retain more control over their health and personal information. A patient record agent could take care of a patient's health data and provide appropriate views only to authorised users to ensure that the integrity of the data is maintained. It would also let the patient know when data are accessed, and by whom.

Patients would be able to authorise health professionals to access their data via their mobile phones, and they could receive updates through wireless technologies, such as Bluetooth. A clinical research agent could help patients who want to participate in research. The agent could find trials for which the patient would be eligible (by checking for patients' specific diagnoses, demographic characteristics, or other inclusion criteria) and notify the researcher without compromising the patient's preferences for privacy or anonymity. In such a case, it might be unclear to a patient's usual GP or specialist whether suitable research was being done, but a software agent programmed to seek out trials for which the patient is eligible opens up new possibilities.

Will clinicians become telecarers?

In the future, health professionals may move towards spending some of their working lives as telecarers. A telecarer is a health professional who delivers responsive, high quality information, services and support to remote patients or clients using the most appropriate communication, such as telephone, email, or instant messaging. The advantages of telecaring include better continuity of care for patients and telecarers being able to work from home some days of the week. Telecaring also brings the need for training and new codes of practice. For example, what responsibility do telecarers have to respond to patient emails promptly, and how do they hand this responsibility over when they go off duty? One health informatics organisation has developed a code of practice for medical use of the internet. The public may even become telecarers for their friends or family, wherever they are—for example, "Dad, will you keep an eye on my diabetes while I'm clubbing in Ibiza?" This raises the question of how much responsibility and information to hand over to patients, parents, or carers. Ultimately, eHealth could allow patients with a chronic disease to club together and set up their own private healthcare organisation in exchange for data (see box opposite).The implications for the local primary care trust or chest physician need to be considered

Concerns about eHealth

Despite its promise for some patients or clinical settings, eHealth technology may not be safe or cost effective. A "plague of pilots" (James Barlow, personal communication, 2004) have

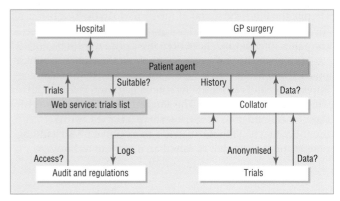

Personal agents could support clinical research. Patients' electronic rights could be represented and protected by their agents. Personal agents could interact on behalf of patients with electronic systems such as web services, databases, and agents representing other individuals, organisations, and functions

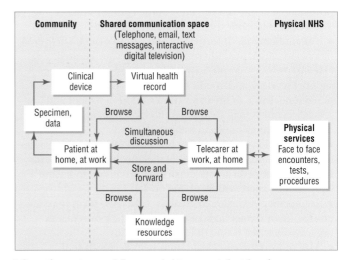

Information systems and flows needed to support the telecaring process

A patient owned healthcare organisation facilitated by the internet

- Asthma patient activists bring together patient organisations and key health professionals as a foundation
- Member patients capture and record data on activity, diet, inhaler use, peak expiratory flow rate, night waking
- The foundation negotiates service contracts for asthma care according to national clinical guidance with GPs, the NHS, and private health providers
- The foundation receives income or free services from health insurers, researchers, or industry in return for data
- This raises the question: who owns patient data—the health system, doctors, or patients? Can the patient give away, sell, or exchange their data for membership of an independent healthcare foundation?

been done, but systematic reviews have shown the evidence about the cost effectiveness of eHealth and telemedicine is poor. It is not clearly understood how telephone triage services influence the use of primary care or emergency services. When triage services go online, changes in demand for health care will follow, but how will emergency and routine services be affected?

Purchases made on credit cards and supermarket loyalty cards could be linked with mobile phones and health records (containing a person's genetic profile) to generate individualised lifestyle advice. But when people are in the supermarket, do they want text messages warning them to avoid fatty food and cut down on alcohol?

Computers can make control of data easier because clinicians can give the encryption key to individual patients. This could allow some people to opt out of the NHS altogether, or only make their data available to clinicians in the NHS for the duration of the consultation. To support quality improvement, health surveillance, and research activities, a compromise between the libertarian position ("it's my data and you can only use it for the period that I say") and a free-for-all must be found.

eHealth has implications for the education, training, and supervision of health professionals. Support will be needed to become a telecarer, and organisations need to explore the implications of substituting telecare for face to face consultations. New ethical and legal issues will arise

The internet has always stood up for individuality, competition, and freedom. Surely a wider market for health services, information, and products should be welcomed? However, if the internet means that commercial suppliers can influence (or mislead) patients, or that "cyber physicians" can undercut physical primary healthcare services, whether and how to regulate eHealth must be considered.

The "cyber divide" worries many policy makers. People with lower educational achievement or income have worse health. They also make less use of the internet. If more healthcare services are shifted to new media, will health inequalities worsen? Interactive digital television is a promising way to reach these communities. The cyber divide also includes the senses— older people rarely use the telephone NHSDirect service, perhaps because of deafness. A web chat alternative has been piloted, and it was appreciated by elderly people, but it seemed too slow to roll out nationally.

Given some of these concerns, people may rise up en masse and reject the use of such technologies in health care, leading to a "Great Revulsion" (Muir Gray, personal communication, 2000), by analogy with the anti-genetically modified foods campaign (see an eHealth nightmare box above).

Summary

The balance of benefits and risks of eHealth for individual patients and clinicians over the next two to three years is unclear. Healthcare organisations and policy makers need to consider the issues that will arise. In the long term, eHealth offers many opportunities for prevention, choice, home based care, and chronic disease management, and it will widen access to health care for most patients. We all need to join the discussion and decide what we want for the future before others, who could be guided by commercial motives rather than quality and equity, do so.

> GPs already feel the "Monday pressure" of health scares that are carried in the Sunday papers. Might rumours from the internet overwhelm the health system?

An eHealth nightmare

Consumer choice and a plethora of commercial eHealth providers lead to multiple, fragmented patient records and supplier-dominated services. There is no single patient identifier or even disease coding system. This results in a health system that cannot access much patient data, and NHS records that hold only a fraction of what is out there. Poor or elderly people feel ever more disconnected from the high tech National eHealth Service. As a result, no National eHealth Service provider can offer a patient centred service. Health scare stories and urban myths spread across the internet like viruses with uncontained fears about privacy, safety and fragmentation of care affecting even cautious patients. Society, led by the media, starts to see technology as inhuman and eHealth becomes the scapegoat (as occurred with genetically modified foods). This leads to eHealth and electronic patient records being rejected by the middle classes, with substitution by a conservative "Holistic health service" emphasising face to face contact and individual freedom of choice—for those who can afford it.

Acknowledgement: Muir Gray

Further reading

- Foresight Health Care Panel. *Healthcare 2020*. London: Department of Trade and Industry, 2000
- Gustafson DH, Wyatt JC. Evaluation of ehealth systems and services. *BMJ* 2004;328:1150
- Borowitz S, Wyatt J. The origin, content and workload of electronic mail consultations. *JAMA* 1998;280:1321-4
- Wyatt JC. The telecarer: a new role for health professionals. In: Lissauer R, Kendall E (eds). *New practitioners in the future health service*. London: Institute for Public Policy Research, 2002
- eHealth code of ethics: www.ihealthcoalition.org/ethics/ethics.html (accessed 28 November 2005)
- Bessell TL, McDonald S, Silagy CA, Anderson JN, Hiller JE, Sansom LN. Do Internet interventions for consumers cause more harm than good? A systematic review. *Health Expect* 2002;5:28-37
- Whitten PS, Mair FS, Haycox A, May CR, Williams TL, Hellmich S. Systematic review of cost effectiveness studies of telemedicine interventions. *BMJ* 2002;324:1434-7
- Turner R. Big brother is looking after your health. *BMJ* 1993;307:1623-4
- Rigby M, Forsström J, Roberts R, Wyatt JC. Verifying quality and safety in health informatics services. *BMJ* 2001;323:552-6
- Eminovic N, Wyatt JC, Tarpey AM, Murray G, Ingrams GJ. First evaluation of the NHS Direct Online Clinical Enquiry Service: A Nurse-led Web Chat Triage Service for the Public. *J Med Internet Res* 2004;6:E17

Glossary

Algorithm
A process for carrying out a complex task broken down into simple decision and action steps. Often assists the *requirements analysis* process carried out before programming.

Bioinformatics
The use of *health informatics* methods to aid or facilitate research in molecular biology.

Checklist
A type of *clinical decision tool*. It is a form listing one or more items of *patient data* to be collected before, during, or after an encounter; can be paper or computer based.

Clinical coding system (clinical thesaurus, controlled vocabulary)
A limited list of preferred terms from which the user can draw one or more to express a concept such as *patient data*, a disease, or drug name. An alphanumeric code corresponding to the term is then stored by the computer. Synonyms or close matches to each preferred term are usually available, and map onto the same internal codes. This approach makes it easier for a computer to analyse data than the use of free text words or phrases. Examples of clinical coding systems include SNOMED-CT (divergent codes used to capture *patient data*), MeSH (terms used to index biomedical literature) and ICD-10 (convergent codes for international comparisons, with specific rules to guide coders). Clinical coding systems play a key role in epidemiological studies and health service research, from the use of MeSH terms to conduct literature searches for systematic reviews to numerous studies which use ICD codes to classify and compare diseases. To prevent information loss, it is vital that the terms and codes are never changed or dropped, only added to. Obsolete terms can be marked as such to deter inappropriate use. Continuing maintenance is needed to incorporate new terms and codes for new concepts and new synonyms as they arise.

Clinical data system
Any information system concerned with the capture, processing, or communication of *patient data*.[1]

Clinical decision tool
Any mechanical, paper or electronic aid that collects data from an individual patient to generate output that aids clinical decisions during the doctor-patient encounter.[2] Examples include *decision support systems*, paper or computer *reminders*, and *checklists*. These are potentially useful tools in *public health informatics*, as well as other branches of health informatics.

Clinical information
Organised *patient data* or *clinical knowledge* used to make clinical decisions (adapted from Shortliffe and colleagues[3]); may also include *directory information*. Many activities in public health and epidemiology (for example, surveillance systems, cohort studies to assess the effects of a risk factor of disease, and clinical trials to estimate efficacies of new treatments) involve the organisation of such data (for example, case report forms for individual patients) into useable information (for example, incidence of notifiable cases of disease from surveillance programmes and summary evidence from cohort studies or clinical trials expressed as odds ratios for certain harmful and beneficial outcomes). See also: *information*.

Clinical informatics
The use of *health informatics* methods to aid management of patients, employing an interdisciplinary approach, including the clinical and information sciences.[3]

Communication
The exchange of *information* between agents (human or automated) face to face or using paper or electronic media.[4] Requires the use of a shared language and understanding or common ground.

Computer vision (image interpretation)
The use of computer techniques to assist the interpretation of images, such as mammograms.

Confidentiality (protecting privacy)
The policies restricting access to a person's data to those whom the patient agrees need access to it, except rarely in emergency and for the public good (for example, to contain epidemics, allow important research to be undertaken or solve serious crime). In addition, other regulatory and institutional approval may be needed (for example, the need to seek consent from medical ethics committees or relevant national authorities). In recent years, leading public health researchers have warned that legislation enacted to protect patients' medical data in the United Kingdom, Europe, and United States could potentially hamper observational research and medical record linkage studies.[5,6]

Consumer health informatics
The use of *health informatics* methods to facilitate the study and development of paper and electronic systems which support public access to and the use of health and lifestyle information. For additional discussion on the scope of consumer health informatics, see Eysenbach.[7] See also: *eHealth*.

Data quality
The degree to which data items are accurate, complete, relevant, timely, sufficiently detailed, appropriately represented (for example, consistently coded using a *clinical coding system*), and retain sufficient contextual information to support decision making.

Database
A collection of data in machine readable format organised so that it can be retrieved or processed automatically by computer. A flat file database is organised like a card file with many records (cards), each including one or more fields (data items). A relational database is organised as one or more related tables, each containing columns and rows. Data are organised in a database according to a schema or data model; some items are often coded using a *clinical coding system*.

Glossary

Decision support system (computer decision aid)

A type of *clinical decision tool*: a computer system that uses two or more items of *patient data* to generate advice for a specific case or encounter.[8] Examples include computer risk assessors to estimate cardiovascular disease risk[9] and the Leeds acute abdominal pain system, which aids the diagnosis of conditions causing such pain.[10] Evidence-adaptive decision support systems are a type of decision aid with a knowledge base that is constructed from and continually adapts to new research- and practice-based evidence.[11]

Decision tree

A way to model a complex decision process as a tree with branches representing all possible intermediate states or final outcomes of an event. The probabilities of each intermediate state or final outcome and the perceived utilities of each are combined to attach expected utilities to each outcome. The science of drawing decision trees and assessing utilities is called decision analysis.

Directory information

Information specific to an organisation or service that is useful in managing public health services, healthcare services, or patients. Examples include a phone directory, a laboratory handbook listing available tests and tubes to use, and a list of the drugs in the local formulary.

eHealth

The use of internet technology by the public, health workers, and others to access health and lifestyle information, services, and support; it encompasses *telemedicine, telecare*. For in-depth discussion on the scope and security issues of eHealth, see report by National HealthKey Collaborative.[12]

Electronic health record (EHR)

In the United Kingdom, the lifelong summary of a person's health episodes, assembled from summaries of individual *electronic patient records* and other relevant data.[13]

Electronic patient record (EPR)

A computer-based *clinical data system* designed to replace paper patient records.

Evaluating health information systems

Measuring or describing the key characteristics of an information system, such as its quality, usability, accuracy, clinical impact, or cost effectiveness.[14] Generally, information systems can be evaluated using standard health technology assessment methods.

Explicit knowledge

Knowledge that can be communicated on paper or electronically, without person-to-person contact.[15] Health workers and physicians cannot use explicit knowledge if they cannot access it. Thus, there is a need to identify, capture, index, and make available explicit knowledge to professionals, a process called codification. Much of the work done by the Cochrane Collaboration involves codification of explicit knowledge. See also: *tacit knowledge*.

Geographical information system (GIS)

Computer software which captures, stores, processes, and displays location as well as other data. The display may preserve distance ratios between data objects (for example, true scale maps) or link similar objects, ignoring distance (for example, topological maps such as that distributed to the

public for the London Underground). GIS software is used in many ecological studies of disease. A famous example is Peto's study of diet, mortality, and lifestyle in rural China.[16] Disease mapping studies have also been conducted to assess childhood leukaemia in areas with different radon levels,[17] the clustering of respiratory cancer cases in areas with a steel foundry[18] and socio-economic gradients in infant mortality.[19] GISs are also used for public health planning and surveillance purposes at local or national health departments. Care should be taken by policy makers in interpreting maps produced by GIS software, particularly in regard to the ecologic fallacy.[20]

Health informatics (medical informatics)

The study and application of methods to improve the management of *patient data, medical knowledge*, population data, and other *information* relevant to patient care and community health. Unlike some other definitions of health or medical informatics (for example, Greens and Shortliffe[21]), this definition puts the emphasis on information management rather than technology. Branches of health informatics include *bioinformatics, clinical informatics, consumer health informatics*, and *public health informatics*.

Information

Organised data or knowledge used by human and computer agents to reduce uncertainty, take decisions and guide actions (adapted from Shortliffe and colleagues[3] and Wyatt[22]). See also: *clinical information, patient data, medical knowledge*.

Information design

The science and practice of designing forms, reports, and books so that the *information* they contain can be found rapidly and interpreted without error (adapted from Sless[23]). Information design is based on psychological and graphical design theories and many empirical studies of human perception and decision making using alternative formats for *information*.

Knowledge base

A store of knowledge (represented explicitly so that a computer can search and reason with it automatically) that often uses a *clinical coding system* to label the concepts. See also: *decision support system*.

Knowledge based system (expert system)

A computer *decision support system* with an explicit *knowledge base* and separate reasoner program. It is used to give advice or interpret data, often *patient data*.

Knowledge management

The identification, mobilisation, and use of knowledge to improve decisions and actions. In public health and medicine much of this work involves the management of *medical knowledge* (from epidemiological studies, randomised-controlled trials and systematic reviews) so that it is used by the physician. This entails clinical practice *innovation*[24] or narrowing the gap between what we know and what we do. The NHS is developing a programme of knowledge codification to inform routine problem solving—for example, through the National Electronic Library of Health, guidelines from the National Institute of Clinical Excellence (NICE), and care pathways and triage algorithms used in the NHS Direct Clinical Advice System.[25]

Medical knowledge (clinical knowledge)

Information about diseases, therapies, interpretation of laboratory tests, and potentially applicable to decisions about multiple patients and public health policies (unlike *patient data*). This information should, where possible, be based on sound evidence from clinical and epidemiological studies, using valid and reliable methods. See also: *explicit knowledge, tacit knowledge, knowledge management*.

Minimum data set

A list of the names, definitions and sources of data items needed to support a specific purpose, such as surveillance of the health of a community, investigation of a research hypothesis or monitoring the quality of care in a *registry*.

Patient data

Information about an individual patient and potentially relevant to decisions about his or her current or future health or illness. Patient data should be collected using methods that minimise systematic and random error. See also: *medical knowledge*.

Public health informatics

The use of *health informatics* methods to promote "public health practice, research and learning," employing an interdisciplinary approach, including the public health sciences (for example, epidemiology and health services research) and the information sciences (for example, computing science and technology) (adapted from Yasnoff and colleagues[26]). In a recent paper outlining an agenda for developing this branch of informatics, Yasnoff and colleagues[27] argued for the need to construct, implement, and integrate public health surveillance systems at national and local level, to enable rapid identification and response to disease hotspots (and more topically, bioterrorism). As Yasnoff points out, methods of assessing costs and benefits of such systems are needed. Public health informatics can also contribute in other areas—for example, reminders have played an important role in prevention programmes such as smoking cessation advice to smokers[28] and the use of preventive care for patients.[29]

Registry

A *database* and associated applications which collects a *minimum data set* on a specified group of patients (often those with a certain disease or who have undergone a specific procedure), health professionals, organisations or even clinical trials. Registries can be used to explore and improve the quality of care or to support research—for example, to monitor long term outcomes or rare complications of procedures. Key issues in registries are maintaining *confidentiality*, coverage of the target population and *data quality*.

Reminder

A type of *clinical decision tool* which reminds a doctor about some item of *patient data* or *clinical knowledge* relevant to an individual patient that they would be expected to know. Can be paper- or computer-based; includes *checklists*, sticky labels on front of notes, an extract from a guideline placed inside notes or computer-based alerts. There has been much interest in reminders as an *innovation method* recently because of the poor uptake of practice guidelines, even those based on good quality evidence. An example is in the treatment of dyslipidaemia in primary care, where there is a big gap between recommendations and actual practice.[30]

Requirements analysis

The process of understanding and capturing user needs, skills, and wishes before developing an information system (adapted from Somerville[31]). See: *software engineering*.

Security

The technical methods by which *confidentiality* is achieved.[12]

Software engineering

The process of system development, documentation, implementation, and upgrading (adapted from Somerville[31]). In the classical or "waterfall" model of software engineering, *requirements analysis* leads to a document that serves as the basis for a system specification and *database* schema, from which programmers work to develop the software. However, increasingly, users and software designers work together from the start to develop and refine a prototype system. This helps to engage the users, educate the software development team, brings the requirements documents alive and allows users to explore how their requirements might change due to interaction with the new software.

Tacit knowledge (intuition)

Knowledge that requires person-to-person contact to transfer and cannot be communicated on paper or electronically.[15,25] Over time, some tacit knowledge can be analysed, decomposed and made explicit. See also: *explicit knowledge*.

Telecare

A kind of *telemedicine* with the patient located in the community (for example, their own home). See also: *eHealth*.

Telemedicine

The use of any electronic medium to mediate or augment clinical consultations. Telemedicine can be simultaneous (for example, telephone, videoconference) or store and forward (for example, an email with an attached image).

Additional resources: Readers who are interested in general coverage of the field of health informatics are encouraged to refer to standard texts.[32,33] Those who are interested in alternative or complementary definitions of the above terms can look up various sources.[3,4,34–36]

Notes to the list of concepts: *Italic* means "see also". Synonyms are mentioned in parentheses, after the core term.

Acknowledgements

Joe Liu, Centre for Statistics in Medicine, Oxford contributed many definitions to an earlier version of this glossary and Ameen Abu Hanna, KIK, AMC Amsterdam provided useful comments.

References

1. Wyatt JC. Clinical data systems I: data and medical records. *Lancet* 1994;344:1543–7
2. Liu JLY, Wyatt JC, Altman DG. *Exploring the definition and scope of clinical decision tools: focus on the problem, not the solution.* Working paper, Centre for Statistics in Medicine, Oxford University, 2002
3. Shortliffe EH, Perreault LE, Wiederhold G, Fagan K. Glossary. In: *Medical informatics—computer applications in health care and biomedicine.* New York: Springer-Verlag, 2001:749–820
4. Van Bemmel JH, Musen M. Glossary. In: *A handbook of medical informatics.* Heidelberg: Springer-Verlag, 1997:557–603
5. Lawlor DA, Stone T. Public health and data protection: an inevitable collision or potential for a meeting of minds. *Int J Epidemiol* 2001;30:1221–5
6. Walton J, Doll R, Asscher W, Hurley R, Langman M, Gillon R, et al. Consequences for research if use of anonymised patient data breaches confidentiality. *BMJ* 1999;319:1366

7. Eysenbach G. Consumer health informatics. *BMJ* 2000;320:1713–6

8. Wyatt JC, Spiegelhalter D. Field trials of medical decision aids: potential problems and solutions. *Proc Ann Symp Comput Applications Med Care* 1991;3–7

9. Hingorani AD, Vallance P. A simple computer programme for guiding management of cardiovascular risk factors and prescribing. *BMJ* 1999;318:101–5

10. Adams ID, Chan M, Clifford PC, Cooke WM, Dallos V, de Dombal FT, et al. Computer aided diagnosis of acute abdominal pain: a multicentre study. *BMJ* 1986;318:101–5

11. Sim I, Gorman P, Robert A, Greenes RA, Haynes RB, Kaplan B, et al. Clinical decision support systems for the practice of evidence-based medicine. *J Am Med Inf Assoc* 2001;8:527–34

12. National HealthKey Collaborative. Securing the exchange and use of electronic health information to improve the nation's health: a summary report to the community. The Robert Wood Johnson Foundation, 2001

13. Burns F. *Information for health.* Leeds: NHS Executive, 1998

14. Friedman CP, Wyatt JC. *Evaluation methods in medical informatics.* New York: Springer-Verlag, 1997

15. Wyatt JC. Management of explicit and tacit knowledge. *J Royal Soc Med* 2001;94:6–9

16. Chen J, Campbell TC, Li J, Peto R. *Diet, lifestyle and mortality in China.* Oxford: Oxford University Press, 1990

17. Kohli S, Brage HN, Lofman O. Childhood leukaemia in areas with different radon levels: a spatial and temporal analysis using GIS. *J Epidemiol Community Health* 2000;54:822–6

18. Lloyd OL. Respiratory-cancer clustering associated with localised industrial air pollution. *Lancet* 1978;1:318–20

19. Wong TW, Wong SL, Yu TS, Liu JLY, Lloyd OL. Socio-economic correlates of infant mortality in Hong Kong using ecologic data 1979–1993. *Scand J Soc Med* 1998;26:281–8

20. Richards TB, Croner CM, Rushton G, Brown CK, Fowler L. Geographic information systems and public health: mapping the future. *Public Health Rep* 1999;114:359–73

21. Greens RA, Shortliffe EH. Medical informatics: an emerging academic discipline and institutional priority. *JAMA* 1990;263:1114–20

22. Wyatt JC. Medical informatics: artefacts or science? *Methods Inf Med* 1996;35:197–200

23. Sless D. What is information design? In: *Designing information for people.* Sydney: Communications Research Press, 1994:1–16

24. Wyatt JC. Practice guidelines and other support for clinical innovation. *J R Soc Med* 2000;93:299–304

25. Wyatt JC. *Clinical knowledge and practice in the information age: a handbook for health professionals.* London: Royal Society of Medicine Press, 2001

26. Yasnoff WA, O'Carroll PW, Koo D, Linkins RW, Kilbourne EM. Public health informatics: improving and transforming public health in the information age. *J Public Health Manage Pract* 2000;6:67–75

27. Yasnoff WA, Overhage JM, Humphreys BL, LaVenture M. A national agenda for public health informatics. *J Am Med Inform Assoc* 2001;8:535–45

28. Law M, Tang JL. An analysis of the effectiveness of interventions intended to help people stop smoking. *Arch Intern Med* 1995;155:1933–41

29. Dexter PR, Perkins S, Overhage JM, Maharry K, Kohler RB, McDonald CJ. A computerized reminder system to increase the use of preventive care for hospitalized patients. *N Engl J Med* 2001;345:965–70

30. Monkman D. Treating dyslipidaemia in primary care: the gap between policy and reality is large in the UK. *BMJ* 2000;321:1299–300

31. Somerville I. *Software engineering,* 5th ed. Wokingham: Addison-Wesley, 1995

32. Wiederhold G, Shortliffe E, Fagan L, Perrault L (eds). *Medical informatics—computer applications in health care and biomedicine.* New York: Springer-Verlag, 2001

33. Coiera E. *Guide to health informatics,* 2nd ed. New York: Chapman and Hall, 2003

34. Bergus GR, Cantor SB, Ebell MH, Ganiats TG, Glasziou PP, Hagan MD, et al. A glossary of medical decision making terms. *Prim Care* 1995;22:385–93

35. Coiera E. Glossary. In: *Guide to health informatics,* 2nd ed. New York: Chapman and Hall, 2003:339–50

36. Hammond E. Glossary for healthcare standards. http://dmi-www.mc.duke.edu/dukemi/acronyms.htm, 1995

Index

abstracts, structured 26
anatomical terms 13
anonymisation of data 31–2
anonymity, collusion of 23, 34
answers, source 26–7
antenatal care, integrated 23
ATTRACT question answering service 14, 26
audio recordings of consultations 15, 21, 23
audit reports 27
automatic query construction 14

Bayes' nomogram 10
Binley's directory information store 33, 34
biometric confidentiality methods 6
biometric sensing devices 16
blood pressure, ambulatory monitoring 9, 17
booking, electronic 17, 22–3, 36

Caldicott Guardians 31
call-recall system 23
cancer registry 13
care
    continuity 21
    data collection 31
    emergency 31
    improvement 24, 29–30
    shared 23
carers 37
case-based reasoning 14
CATmaker 27
CD-Roms of books 17
checklists 7
choose and book 32
chronic care model 23
classification of data 9, 20
clinical data 2–3
    accessing 17
    accuracy 21
    anonymisation 31
    classification 9, 20
    coding 9, 20
    completeness 21
    confidential sources 9
    confidentiality 31
    criteria for quality 3
    direct 9
    feedback 29–30
    integration 24, 29
    interpretation 29
    presentation 29
    quality 3, 19
    record linkage 30
    recording 21
    routine extraction 30
    secondary uses 20, 29
    security 31

sources 29
    structured recording 20
    see also medical records
clinical decisions
    making 18
    rules 20–1
    support tools 11
clinical enquiry forms 36
clinical evidence resource 26
clinical governance 2, 24
    definition 29
clinical information 1
    capturing 1–2
    carers 36
    electronic systems 12
    exchange 33
    feedback 31
    gathering/recording during consultation 19–20
    quality 3
    resource availability for patients 17
    sharing 23
    sources 2–3, 11–12
    using 1–2
clinical knowledge sources 1
clinical practice, changing 30
clinical prediction rules 20–1
clinical questions 25–6, 28
    answering services 14, 26–7
    clear 26
    log books 27
    PubMed search filters 27
clinical research agents 36
clinical trials 37
codes of practice, telecarers 36
coding of data 3, 9, 20
collusion of anonymity 23, 34
communication channels 34
communication of information 1, 32–3
    interactive 13
community health index 12, 30
computers
    in consultation 14–15, 19–21
    handheld 17, 19
    sharing of understanding 13–15
confidential sources of data 9
confidentiality
    clinical data 31
    medical records 20
    teleconsultation 6
consent, explicit/inferred 31
consultation models
    of Pendleton 1
    of Stott and Davies 10
consultations 4–6
    accessing information after 15, 17
    audio recording 15, 21, 23

Index

consultations (*contd.*)
    computers in 14–15, 19–21
    information retrieval 14
    knowledge integration 12
    patient outcomes 13
    patient-centred 23
    reasons for 7–9
    trust 21
continuing problems management 10–11
continuing professional development 25
continuity, organisational 21
costs of information 3
    eHealth 36
    informatics tools 21
critically appraised topics (CAT) 27
cyber divide 37

data
    processing principles 31
    see also clinical data
data protection 31
Data Protection Act (1998) 9, 31
databases 11
    prognostic 14
decision making
    biometric sensing devices 16
    rapid 20
decision support tools 8, 10 12, 13
    software 16
democracy 35
deterministic methods 30
diagnostic process 7
diagrams 13
DIPEX 5
directory information 2, 32–4
diseases, partial hierarchy 3
display of information 2
drug history 8
drug information services 26

early detection of problems 22
economics 36
education *see* medical education; patient
    education
eHealth 4, 35–7
    concerns 37
    development 35–6
    tools 4
electronic prompts 22
    patient problems 10, 11
email 6
    clinical topics 17
    discussion groups 27
    laboratory results 16
    telecarers 36
emergency care 31
empowerment, patient 23
encryption keys 37
ethics, eHealth implications 37
EU directive on data protection
    (1995) 31
evidence, Grade 1 11
evidence-based guidelines 11
expert patients 23

family history 8
follow-up
    arranging 23
    consultations 9
    general practitioners 23
    hospital 23
    level 21

format for information 2
Freedom of Information Act (2000) 31
general practitioners
    eHealth uses 36
    follow-up 23
    telecare 37
    see also primary care

genogram 13
genomics 12
glossary 39–42
good practice, Data Protection Act 31
GP Quality and Outcomes Framework (2004) 11
guidelines 6, 11
    computerised 11
    early detection 22

health biographies 36
health communication, interactive 13
health inequalities 37
health information 1–3
Health Insurance Portability and Accountability Act (US) 31
health maintenance organisations 36
health policy 35
health portals, patient-orientated 4–5
health promotion, opportunistic 10
health records
    effective integration 12
    electronic 12, 14
    see also medical records
HealthSpace 33
healthcare organisations 36
healthcare system navigation 32–4
help seeking behaviour modification 10, 12
hospitals
    admissions data 19
    follow-up 23
    outpatient booking website 17
    see also booking, electronic
human annotation 14
human searchers 14
hypothetico-deductive reasoning 7

icons 2
images 13, 14
inductive reasoning 7
informatics tools 16–18, 21, 29–31
information retrieval
    consultations 14
    multimedia 13–14
    needs 13
    see also clinical information
informed consent 31
insight sharing 27
integrated services 11
interactive cases 27
internet 37
    patient-orientated health portals 4–5
    resources 4
    search engines 4
    see also email; websites; wireless networks
interpretation of information 2
investigations, appropriate 22

Johari window 10
just in time learning 17, 26

knowledge
    accessing 17
    medical 2
    sources 1

laboratory results 8
    email 16

laptops 19
learning in workplace 25–8
  cultural changes 27, 28
  just in time 17, 26
  lifelong, self-directed 26
  motivation 28
  online 27
legal issues, eHealth implications 37
library 28
  workplace 26
Library for Health, electronic 25
lifestyle advice, text messages 37
lifetime risk 13
log books 27

management of patient 19
mediated access 5
Medical Directory 34
medical education 25
  eHealth implications 37
  undergraduate 28
medical history 7–8
medical knowledge 2
medical literature access 5
  CD-Roms of books 17
  mediated 5–6
  see also library; websites
medical records 1
  confidentiality 20
  electronic 8, 11, 12
    clinical governance 24
    compliance with requirements 20
    organisational continuity 21
  integration 12, 24
  linkage 30
  paper 8
  patient access 33
  security 20
  see also clinical data
Medline 26
meta-analyses 11
metabonomics 12
modifying factors, odds ratio 10
motivation, workplace learning 28
multiagent systems 37
multidisciplinary working 27
multimedia, information retrieval 13–14

national programme for information technology (NPfIT) 32
NHS Confederation 34
NHS Direct service 8, 37
  telecarers 36
NHS Healthspace 33, 36
NHS poisons and drug information services 26
nomenclature, medical 20
NPFiT 32
nurses
  telecare 37
  triage 8

odds ratio, modifying factors 10
online learning 27
opportunistic health promotion 10
organisational governance 34
Ottawa ankle rule 20
out-of-hours doctors 31

parochialism 27
paternalism, state 37
patient(s)
  eHealth demand 35
  empowerment 23

encryption keys 37
expert 23
  internet resources 4
  medical literature access 5–6
  responsibility 36
  unique identification system 12
patient education 17
  materials 14
patient problems
  electronic prompts 10, 11
  informatics tools 16–18
  presenting 16
patient simulators 27
Pendleton's consultation model 1
performance data, feedback 29–30
personal agents 36
poisons and drug information services 26
preconsultation screening tools 8
prescribing record 8
prescriptions, repeat 36
presentation giving 27
primary care
  directory information 32
  follow-up 23
  workplace learning 28
  see also general practitioners
probabilistic methods 30
probability 10
problem, intervention, comparison and outcome (PICO) model 26
problem(s)
  early detection 22
  resolving 29
  see also patient problems
problem solving algorithms 8
PRODIGY software 16, 22
prognosis 14
prompts *see* electronic prompts
proteomics 12
protocols 7
PubMed search filters 27
push technology 4, 17

quality assurance, health portals 4, 5
quality of information 3
queries during consultation 14
questionnaires 6
  screening tools 10

randomized controlled trial (RCT) 11
Read data coding system 9
reasoning
  hypothetico-deductive 7
  inductive 7
recurrence risk 21
reference materials 14
  after consultation 15
referral 17
  arranging 22–3
  earlier 22–4
  electronic form 17, 22–3
reflective practice 26
registry information 13
reminders 22
repeat prescribing 8
representation of information 2
research governance 31
responsibility, carers/patients 36
risk
  lifetime 13
  prediction tools 14
  recurrence 21
Risk Assessment in Genetics software (RAGs) 13

Index

safety 35
screening, call-recall system 23
screening tools 10
search by navigation 14
search engines 4
security
   clinical data 31
   medical records 20
semiotic theory 2
shared care 23
smart cards 8
SNOMED data coding system 9, 20
Soundex system 30
state paternalism 37
Stott and Davies consultation model 10
supervision, eHealth implications 37
symptoms checklist 7
systematic reviews 3, 26

teachable moments 26
technology
   developments 35
   rejection 37
telecarers 36

teleconsultation 6
telemetry 16
telephone triage services 37
television, digital 37
text messages, lifestyle advice 37
training
   eHealth implications 37
   telecarers 36
triage nurses 8
triage services 37
trust, consultations 21
Turning Research into Practice (TRIP)
   database 11

video messaging 6

webcams 6
websites 13, 15
   hospital outpatient booking 17
   information exchange/transactions 35
wireless networks 17, 19, 36
workforce 35
workplace learning 27
write once read many 19